The Delicious Anti-Inflammatory Cooking Guide

A Recipe Collection to improve your Anti-Inflammatory Diet

Thomas Jollif

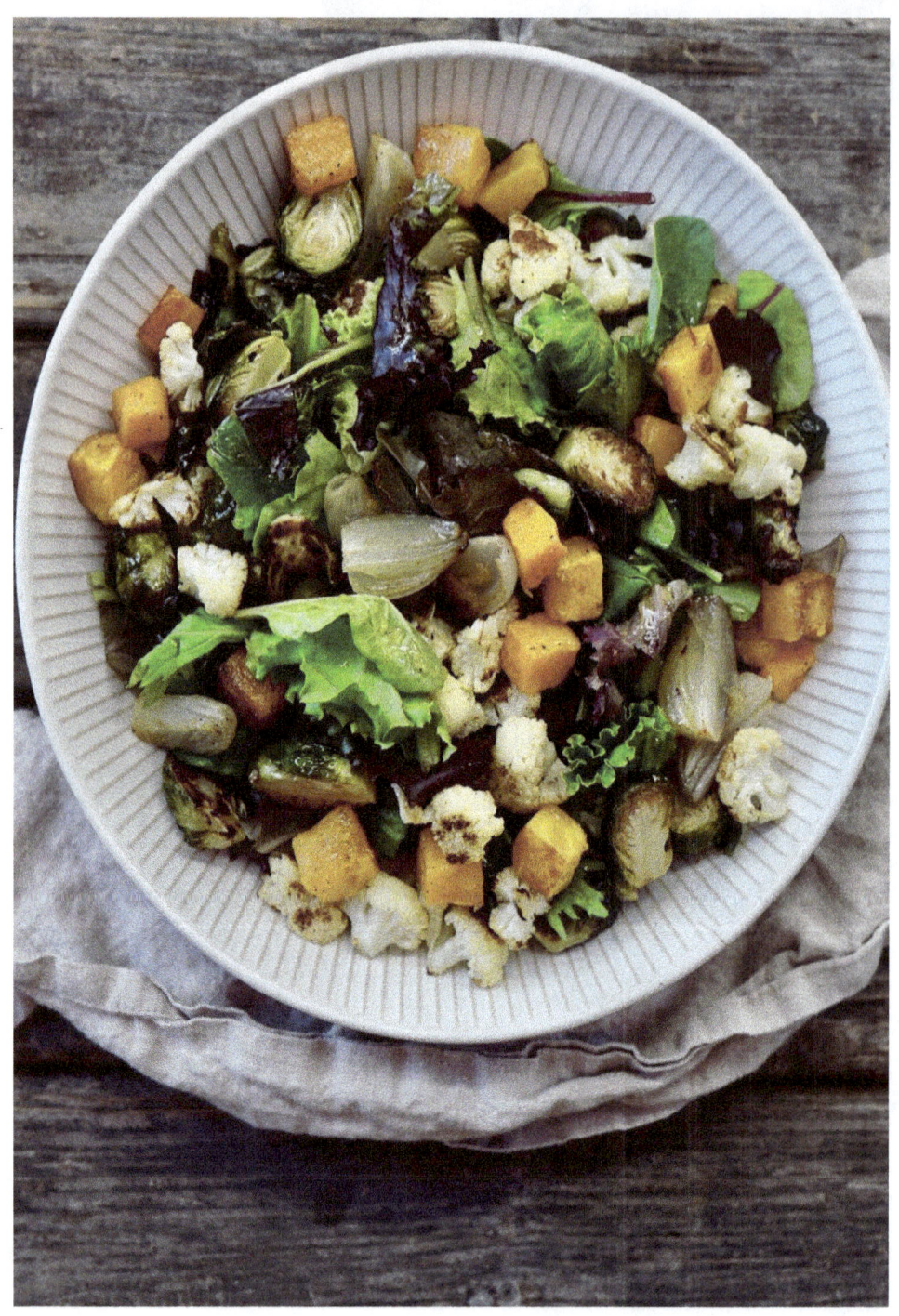

© copyright 2021 – all rights reserved.

the content contained within this book may not be reproduced, duplicated or transmitted without direct written permission from the author or the publisher.

under no circumstances will any blame or legal responsibility be held against the publisher, or author, for any damages, reparation, or monetary loss due to the information contained within this book. either directly or indirectly.

legal notice:

this book is copyright protected. this book is only for personal use. you cannot amend, distribute, sell, use, quote or paraphrase any part, or the content within this book, without the consent of the author or publisher.

disclaimer notice:

please note the information contained within this document is for educational and entertainment purposes only. all effort has been executed to present accurate, up to date, and reliable, complete information. no warranties of any kind are declared or implied. readers acknowledge that the author is not engaging in the rendering of legal, financial, medical or professional advice. the content within this book has been derived from various sources. please consult a licensed professional before attempting any techniques outlined in this book.

by reading this document, the reader agrees that under no circumstances is the author responsible for any losses, direct or indirect, which are incurred as a result of the use of information contained within this document, including, but not limited to, — errors, omissions, or inaccuracies.

Table of Contents

BREAKFASTS 7
Fennel Seeds Cookies 7
Flaxseed Porridge with Cinnamon 9
Fruity Muffins 11
Gingerbread Oatmeal Breakfast 13
Grapefruit-Pomegranate Salad 15
Greek Yogurt with Cherry-Almond Syrup Parfait ... 17
Ham and Veggie Frittata Muffins 19
Hash Browns 22
Honey Pancakes 24
Huevos Rancheros 27

SMOOTHIES AND DRINKS 28
Green Vanilla Smoothie 28
Hibiscus Tea 30
Hot Apple Cider 32
Hot Peppermint Vanilla Latte 34
Instant Horchata 36
Jamaican Hibiscus Tea 37
Kale Smoothie 39
Kiwi Strawberry Smoothie 41

SIDES 43
Lentil Salad 43

MASCARPONE COUSCOUS 45
MOROCCAN STYLE COUSCOUS 46
MUSHROOM MILLET 48

SAUCES AND DRESSINGS 50

CUCUMBER AND DILL SAUCE 50
DAIRY-FREE CREAMY TURMERIC DRESSING 52

SNACKS 54

COTTAGE CHEESE WITH APPLE SAUCE 54
CUCUMBER ROLLS HORS D'OEUVRES 55
CUCUMBER YOGURT 58
DELECTABLE COOKIES 60
DRIED DATES & TURMERIC TRUFFLES 62
EASY GUACAMOLE 64
EASY PEASY GINGER DATE 65

SOUPS AND STEWS 67

GARLIC MUSHROOM & BEEF SOUP 67
GARLICKY CHICKEN SOUP 69
GOLDEN CHICKPEA AND VEGETABLE SOUP 71
GREEK SPLIT PEA SOUP 73
GREEN BLAST SOUP 75
GUT-HEALING BONE BROTH 77
HAMBURGER & TOMATO SOUP 79
HARVEST STEW 81
HEARTY ROOT VEGETABLE SOUP 83

DESSERTS 85

CREAMY & CHILLY BLUEBERRY BITES 85

- CREAMY FROZEN YOGURT 87
- DARK CHOCOLATE GRANOLA BARS 89
- DATE DOUGH & WALNUT WAFER 91
- EASY PEACH COBBLER 94
- FALL-TIME CUSTARD 96
- FENNEL AND ALMOND BITES 98
- FLOURLESS SWEET POTATO BROWNIES 100
- FRIED PINEAPPLE SLICE 102
- FRUIT COBBLER 104

BREAKFASTS

Fennel Seeds Cookies

Time To Prepare: ten minutes
Time to Cook: twenty minutes
Yield: Servings 5

Ingredients:

- ¼ cup coconut oil, softened
- ¼ teaspoon whole fennel seeds
- ½ teaspoon fresh ginger, grated finely
- 1 teaspoon vanilla extract
- 1/3 cup coconut flour
- 2 tablespoons raw honey
- Pinch freshly ground black pepper
- Pinch of ground cinnamon
- Pinch of salt

Directions:

1. Set the oven to 360°F. Coat a cookie sheet that has a parchment paper.
2. In a substantial container, put in all together the ingredients and mix till a uniform dough form.

3. Form a small balls in the mixture make onto a prepared cookie sheet inside a single layer.
4. Using your fingers, softly push along the balls to form the cookies.
5. Bake for minimum 9 minutes or till golden brown.

Nutritional Info: Calories: 353 ‖ Fat: 5g ‖ Carbohydrates: 19g ‖ Fiber: 3g ‖ Protein: 25g

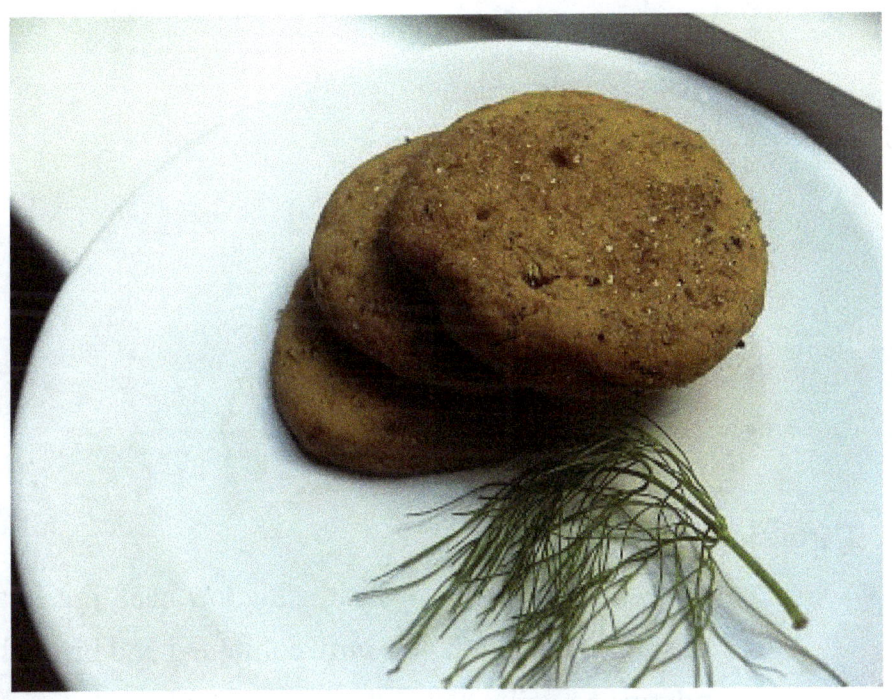

Flaxseed Porridge with Cinnamon

Time To Prepare: ten minutes
Time to Cook: five minutes
Yield: Servings 4

Ingredients:

- ½ cup shredded coconut
- 1 cup heavy cream
- 1 tbsp. unsalted butter
- 1 tsp cinnamon
- 1½ tsp stevia
- 2 cups of water
- 2 tbsp. flaxseed meal
- 2 tbsp. flaxseed oatmeal

Directions:

1. Take a medium pot, place it using low heat, put in all the ingredients in it, stir until combined and bring the mixture to boil.
2. When the mixture has boiled, remove the pot from heat, stir it well and split it uniformly between four bowls.

3. Let porridge rest for about ten minutes until slightly become thick and then serve.

Nutritional Info: Calories 171 ‖ Total Fat: 16g ‖ Carbs: 6g ‖ Protein: 2g

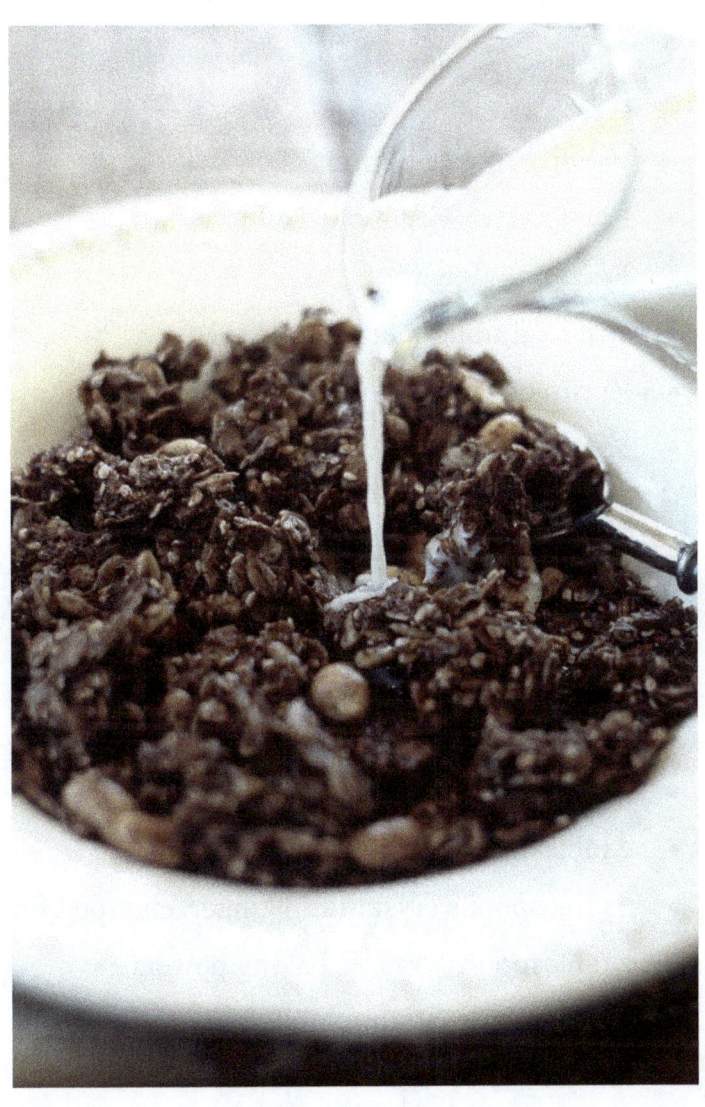

Fruity Muffins

Time To Prepare: ten minutes
Time to Cook: 2-3 minutes
Yield: Servings 8

Ingredients:

- ¼ cup brown rice flour
- ¼ cup extra-virgin olive oil
- ¼ cup raw sugar
- ½ cup almond meal
- ½ cup buckwheat flour
- ½ teaspoon ground ginger
- 1 big organic egg
- 1 cup rhubarb, cut finely
- 1 small apple, peeled, cored and chopped finely
- 1 tablespoon linseed meal
- 1 teaspoon organic vanilla extract
- 12 teaspoon ground cinnamon
- 2 tablespoons arrowroot flour
- 2 tablespoons crystallized ginger, chopped finely
- 2 tablespoons organic baking powder
- 7 tablespoons almond milk
- Pinch of salt

Directions:

1. Set the oven to 350F. Grease 8 cups of a big muffin tin.
2. In a big container, combine almond meal, linseed meal, sugar, and crystalized ginger.
3. In another container, put together flours, baking powder, spices, and salt, and mix.
4. Sift the flour mixture into the container of almond meal mixture and mix thoroughly.
5. In a third container, put in egg, milk, oil, and vanilla and beat till well blended.
6. Put in egg mixture into the flour mixture and mix till well blended.
7. Fold in apple and rhubarb.
8. Put the mixture into prepared muffin cups equally.
9. Bake for approximately 20-twenty-five minutes or till a toothpick inserted in the middle comes out clean.

Nutritional Info: Calories: 227 ‖ Total Fat: 4.2g ‖ Total Carbohydrates: 26.9g ‖ Fiber: 4.9g Sugars: 10.4g ‖ Protein: 4.1g

Gingerbread Oatmeal Breakfast

Time To Prepare: ten minutes
Time to Cook: 0 minutes
Yield: Servings 4

Ingredients:

- ¼ tsp ground allspice
- ¼ tsp ground cardamom
- ¼ tsp ground coriander
- ¼ tsp ground ginger
- 1 ½ tbsp. ground cinnamon
- 1 cup steel-cut oats
- 1 tsp ground cloves
- 1/8 tsp nutmeg
- 4 cups drinking water
- Fresh mixed berries
- Organic Maple syrup, to taste

Directions:

1. Cook the oats based on the package instructions. When it comes to its boiling point, decrease the heat and simmer.

2. Mix in all the spices and carry on cooking until cooked to desired doneness.
3. Serve in four serving bowls and sprinkle with maple syrup and top with fresh berries.
4. Enjoy!

Nutritional Info: Calories: 87 kcal ‖ Protein: 5.82 g ‖ Fat: 3.26 g ‖ Carbohydrates: 18.22 g

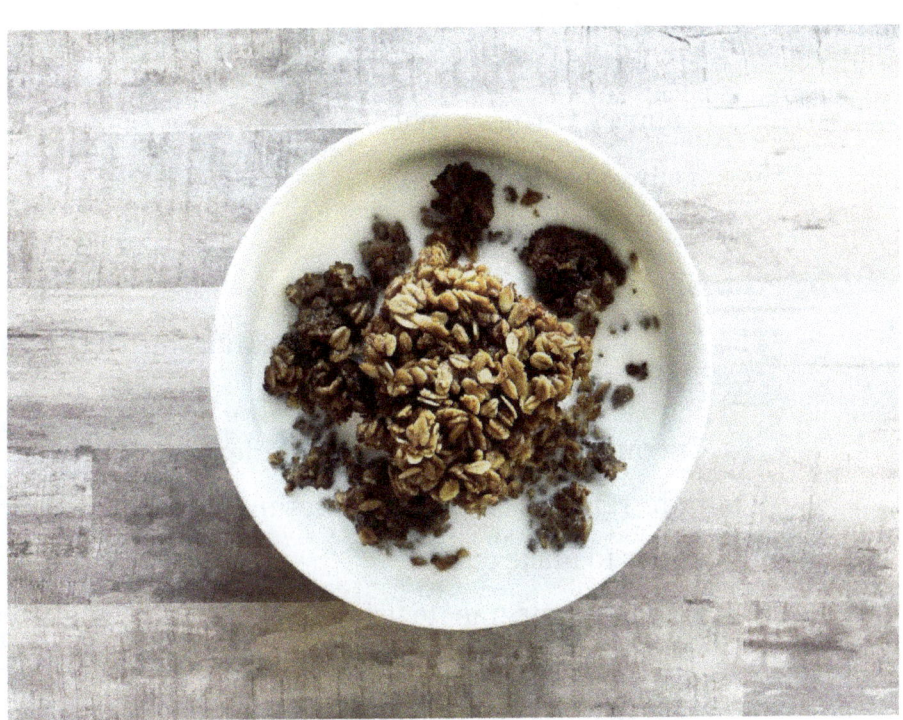

Grapefruit-Pomegranate Salad

Time To Prepare: ten minutes
Time to Cook: 0 minutes
Yield: Servings 6

Ingredients:

- ¼ cup Basic Vegetable Stock
- 1 pomegranate
- 2 ruby red grapefruits
- 3 ounces Parmesan cheese
- 6 cups mesclun leaves

Directions:

1. Peel the grapefruit using a knife, take off all the pith. (the white layer under the skin).
2. Cut out every section with the knife, make sure that no pith remains. Shave Parmesan using a vegetable peeler to make curls.
3. Peel the pomegranate using a paring knife; take off the berries/seeds.
4. Toss the mesclun greens in the stock.
5. To serve, mound the greens on plates and position the grapefruit sections, cheese, and pomegranate on top.

Nutritional Info: Calories: 84 ‖ Fat: 2 g ‖ Protein: 4 g ‖ Sodium: 102 mg ‖ Fiber: 2 g ‖ Carbohydrates: 14 g

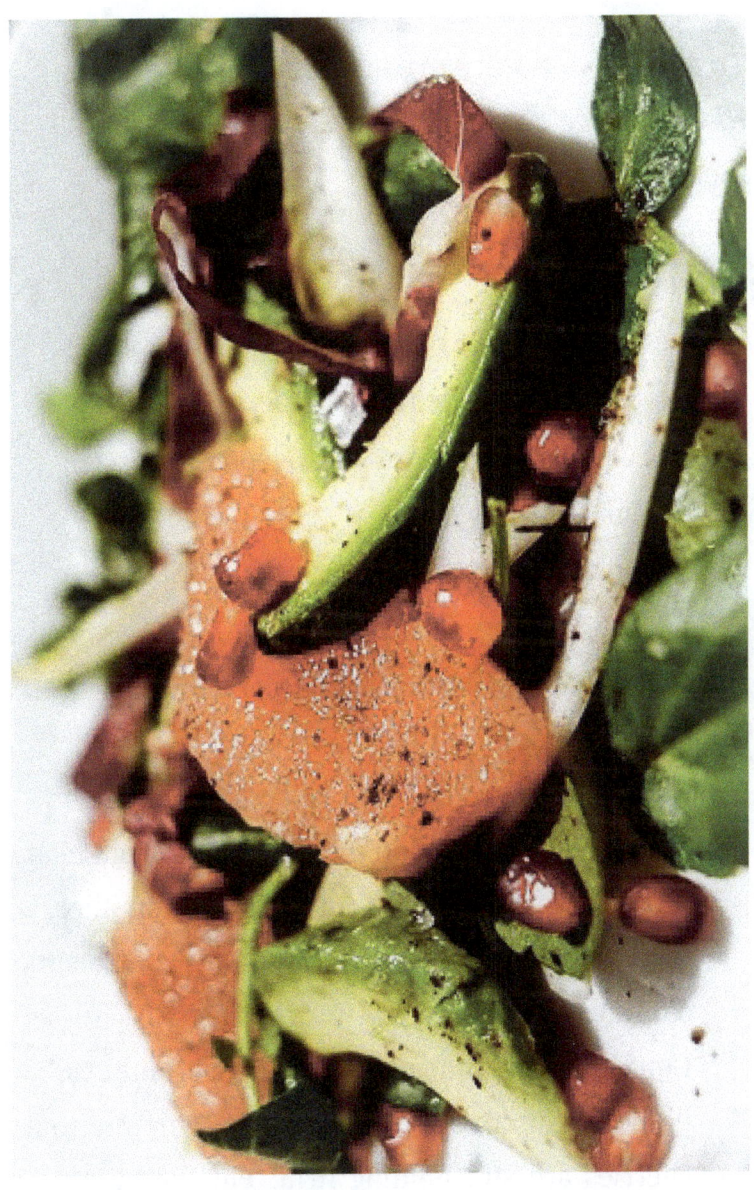

Greek Yogurt with Cherry-Almond Syrup Parfait

Time To Prepare: twenty-five minutes
Time to Cook: five minutes
Yield: Servings 2

Ingredients:

- 1 c. fresh black or red cherries, pitted
- 1 tsp. fresh-squeezed lemon juice
- 2 c. Greek plain yogurt, stir to loosen
- 2 tbsp. almond syrup
- 2 tbsp. coconut palm sugar
- 2 tbsp. cut almonds, to decorate
- 4 tbsp. granola of choice, to decorate (opt.)

Directions:

1. Put a deep cooking pan on moderate to high heat and mix cherries, almond syrup, sugar, lemon juice, and 1 tbsp. of water. Stir to blend, then place it to simmer, continuously stirring until sugar is dissolved. Continue to simmer for further five minutes, until liquid begins to turn into a syrupy mixture, but the cherries are still holding firm. Put the mixture to a

container and allow to cool for five minutes at room temperature, then bring it in your fridge to chill until it is completely cold.
2. Put 1 cup of Greek yogurt into 2 serving bowls and spoon ½ of the cherries and their syrupy juices over the yogurt. Decorate using cut almonds or granola, if you wish. Serve instantly.

Nutritional Info: Calories: 185 kcal ‖ Protein: 4.75 g ‖ Fat: 4.88 g ‖ Carbohydrates: 33.07 g

Ham and Veggie Frittata Muffins

Time To Prepare: ten minutes
Time to Cook: twenty-five minutes
Yield: Servings 12

Ingredients:

- ¼ cup coconut milk (canned)
- ½ yellow onion, finely diced
- 1 cup cherry tomatoes, halved
- 2 tablespoons coconut flour
- 4 tablespoons coconut oil
- 5 ounces thinly cut ham
- 8 big eggs
- 8 oz. frozen spinach, thawed and drained
- 8 oz. mushrooms, thinly cut
- Sea salt and pepper to taste

Directions:

1. Preheat your oven to 375 degrees Fahrenheit.
2. In a moderate-sized frying pan, warm the coconut oil on moderate heat. Put in the onion and cook until tender.

3. Put in the mushrooms, spinach, and cherry tomatoes. Sprinkle with salt and pepper. Cook until the mushrooms have become tender. About five minutes. Turn off the heat and save for later.
4. In a huge container, beat the eggs with the coconut milk and coconut flour. Mix in the cooled the veggie mixture.
5. Coat each cavity of a 12 cavity muffin tin with the thinly cut ham. Pour the egg mixture into each one and bake for about twenty minutes.
6. Take out of the oven and let cool for approximately five minutes before transferring to a wire rack.

Nutritional Info: Calories: 125 kcal ‖ Protein: 5.96 g ‖ Fat: 9.84 g ‖ Carbohydrates: 4.48 g

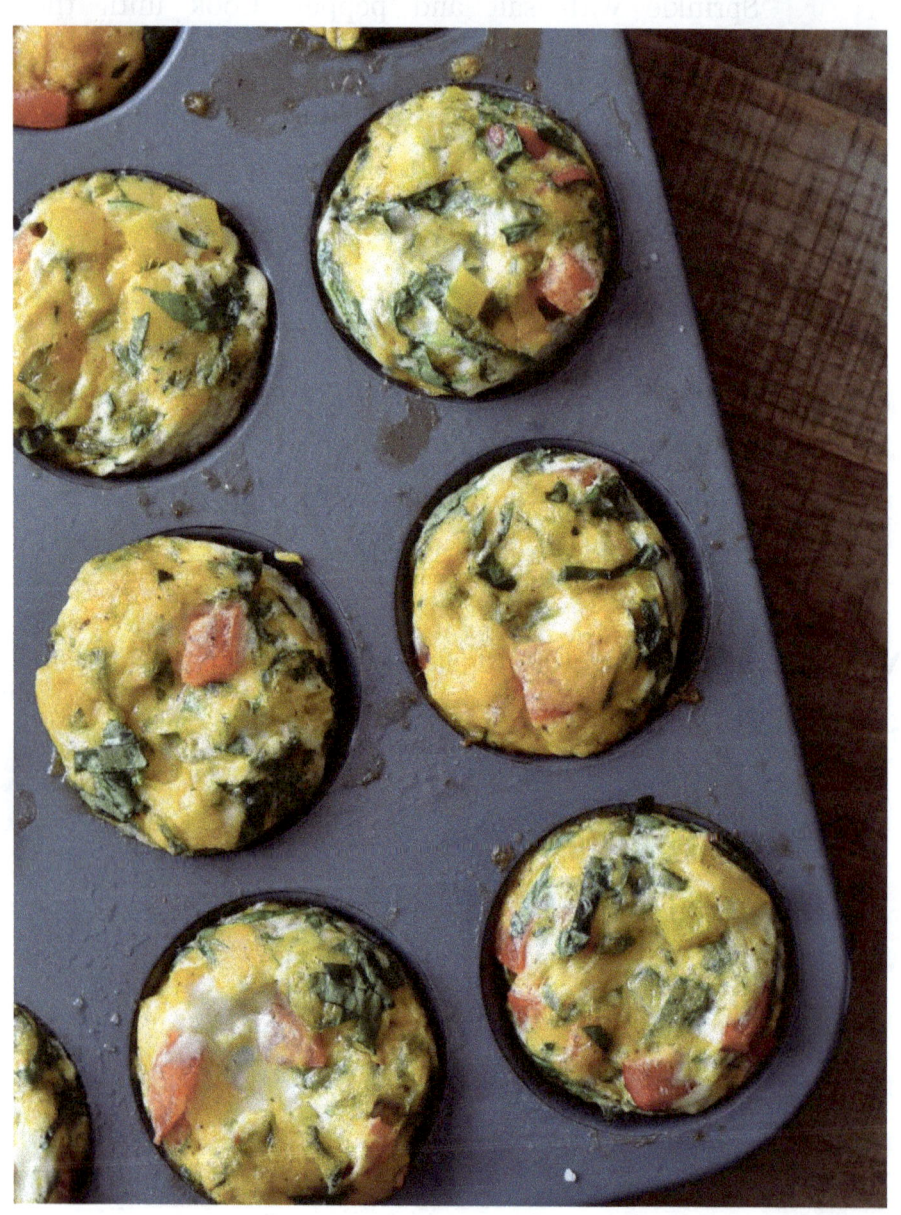

Hash Browns

Time To Prepare: fifteen minutes
Time to Cook: fifteen minutes
Yield: Servings 4

Ingredients:

- 1 pound Russet potatoes, peeled, processed using a grater
- 3 Tbsp. olive oil
- Pinch of black pepper, to taste
- Pinch of sea salt

Directions:

1. Coat a microwave safe-dish using paper towels. Spread shredded potatoes on top. Microwave veggies on the maximum heat setting for a couple of minutes. Turn off the heat.
2. Pour 1 tablespoon of oil into a non-stick frying pan set on moderate heat.
3. Cooking in batches, place a generous pinch of potatoes into the hot oil. Push down using the back of a spatula.
4. Cook for about three minutes every side, or until brown and crunchy. Drain over paper towels. Repeat

step for remaining potatoes. Put in more oil as required.
5. Sprinkle with salt and pepper and serve.

Nutritional Info: Calories: 200 kcal ‖ Protein: 4.03 g ‖ Fat: 11.73 g ‖ Carbohydrates: 20.49 g

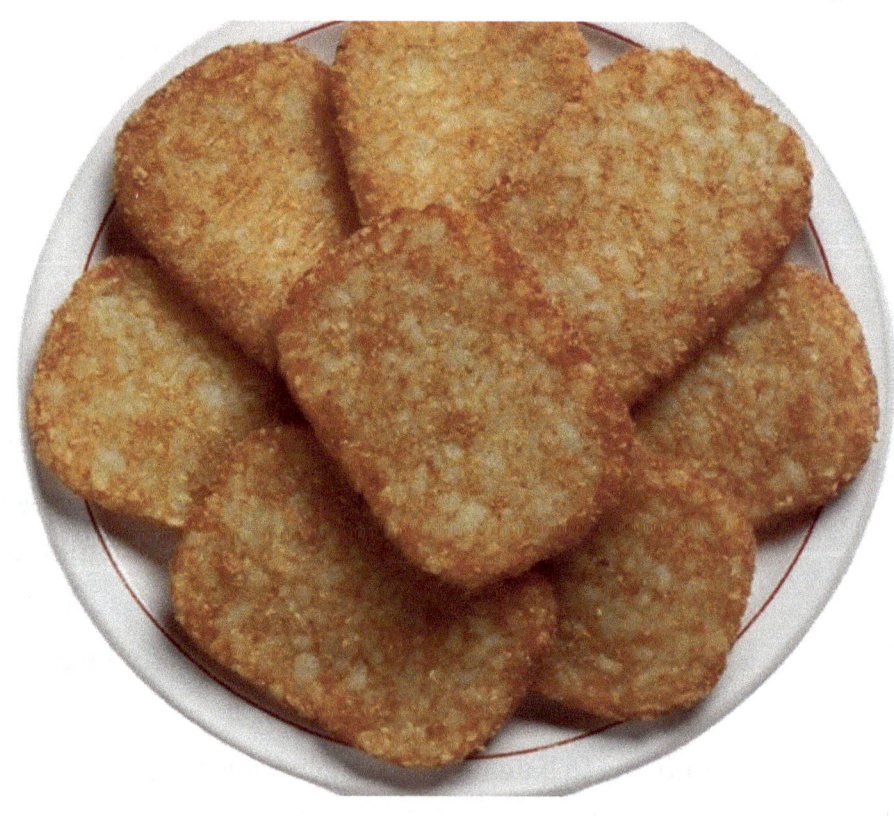

Honey Pancakes

Time To Prepare: ten minutes
Time to Cook: five minutes
Yield: Servings 2

Ingredients:

- ¼ tsp baking soda
- ½ cup almond flour
- ½ tablespoon ground cinnamon
- ½ tablespoon ground ginger
- ½ tablespoon ground nutmeg
- ½ teaspoon ground cloves
- ½ teaspoon organic vanilla extract
- ¾ cup organic egg whites
- 1 tablespoon ground flaxseeds
- 2 tablespoons coconut flour
- 2 tablespoons organic honey
- Coconut oil, as required
- Pinch of salt

Directions:

1. In a big container, combine flours, flax seeds, baking soda, spices, and salt.

2. In another container, put in honey, egg whites and vanilla and beat till well blended.
3. Place the egg mixture into the flour mixture then mix till well blended.
4. Lightly, grease a big nonstick frying pan with oil and heat on medium-low heat.
5. Put in about ¼ cup of mixture and tilt the pan to spread it uniformly inside the frying pan.
6. Cook for approximately 3-4 minutes.
7. Cautiously, customize the side and cook roughly one minute more.
8. Repeat with the rest of the mixture.
9. Serve together with your desired topping.

Nutritional Info: Calories: 291 ‖ Fat: 8g ‖ Carbohydrates: 26g ‖ Fiber: 4g ‖ Protein: 23g

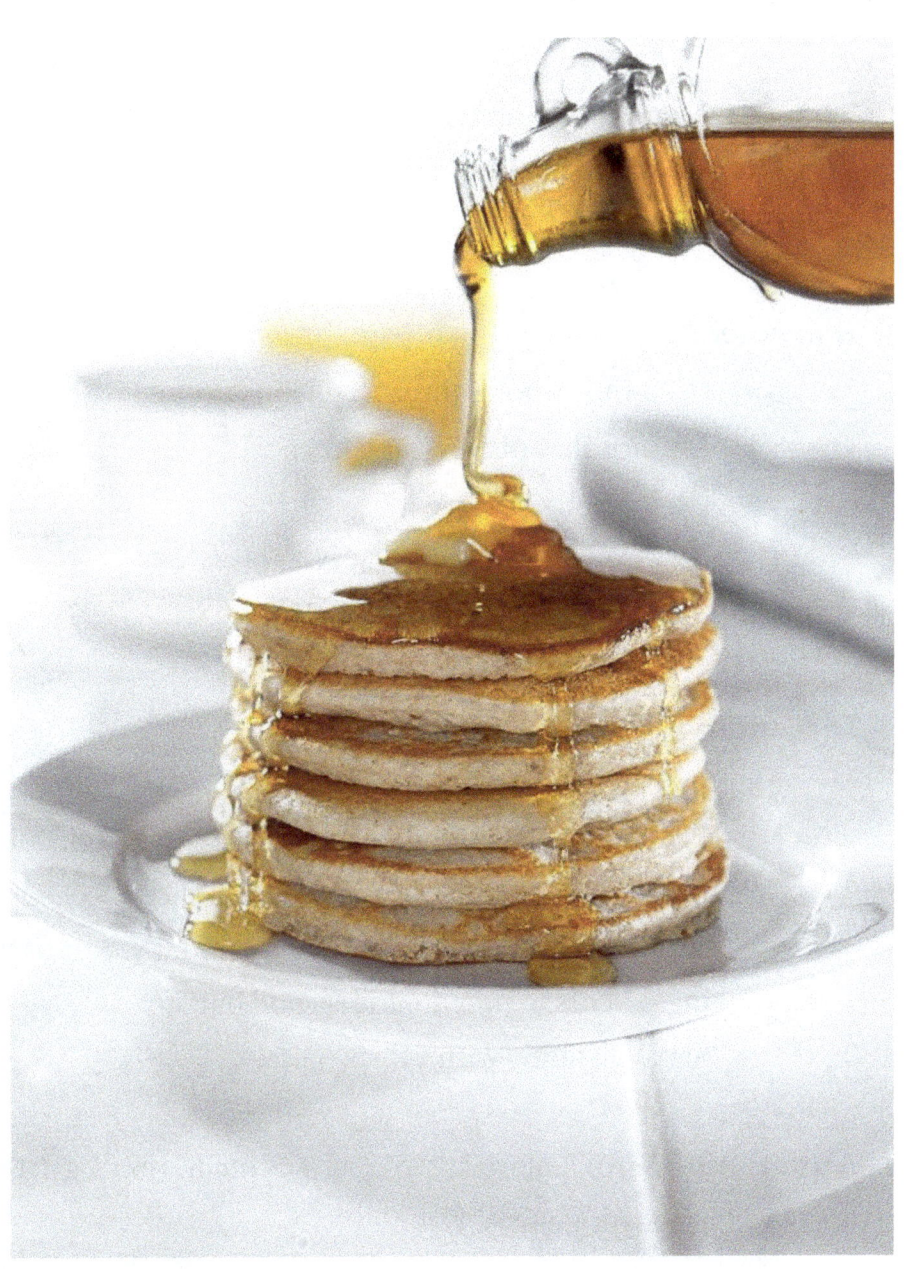

Huevos Rancheros

Time To Prepare: five minutes
Time to Cook: five minutes
Yield: Servings 2

Ingredients:
- (2) 8-inch whole wheat tortillas
- 1-ounce slice of cheddar cheese
- 2 hard-boiled eggs, cut
- 2 slices of Canadian bacon or ham
- 2 tbsp. salsa

Directions:
1. Prepare the hardboiled eggs.
2. Put one tortilla on a plate, top with a slice of Canadian bacon or ham, the cut egg, and a slice of cheddar cheese. Roll the tortilla up. Repeat with the rest of the ingredients to prepare the second burrito.
3. Serve instantly with 1 tbsp. Salsa.

Nutritional Info: Calories: 741 kcal ‖ Protein: 36.12 g ‖ Fat: 30.75 g ‖ Carbohydrates: 79.37 g

SMOOTHIES AND DRINKS

Green Vanilla Smoothie

Time To Prepare: ten minutes
Time to Cook: 0 minutes
Yield: Servings 1

Ingredients:
- 1 1/2 cups fresh spinach leaves
- 1 banana, cut in chunks
- 1 cup grapes
- 1 tub (6 oz.) vanilla yogurt
- 1/2 apple, cored and chopped

Directions:
1. Put in everything to a blender jug.
2. Cover the jug firmly.
3. Blend until the desired smoothness is achieved. Serve and enjoy!

Nutritional Info: Calories: 131 ‖ Fat: 0.2 g ‖ Protein: 2.6 g ‖ Carbohydrates: 9.1 g ‖ Fiber: 1.3 g

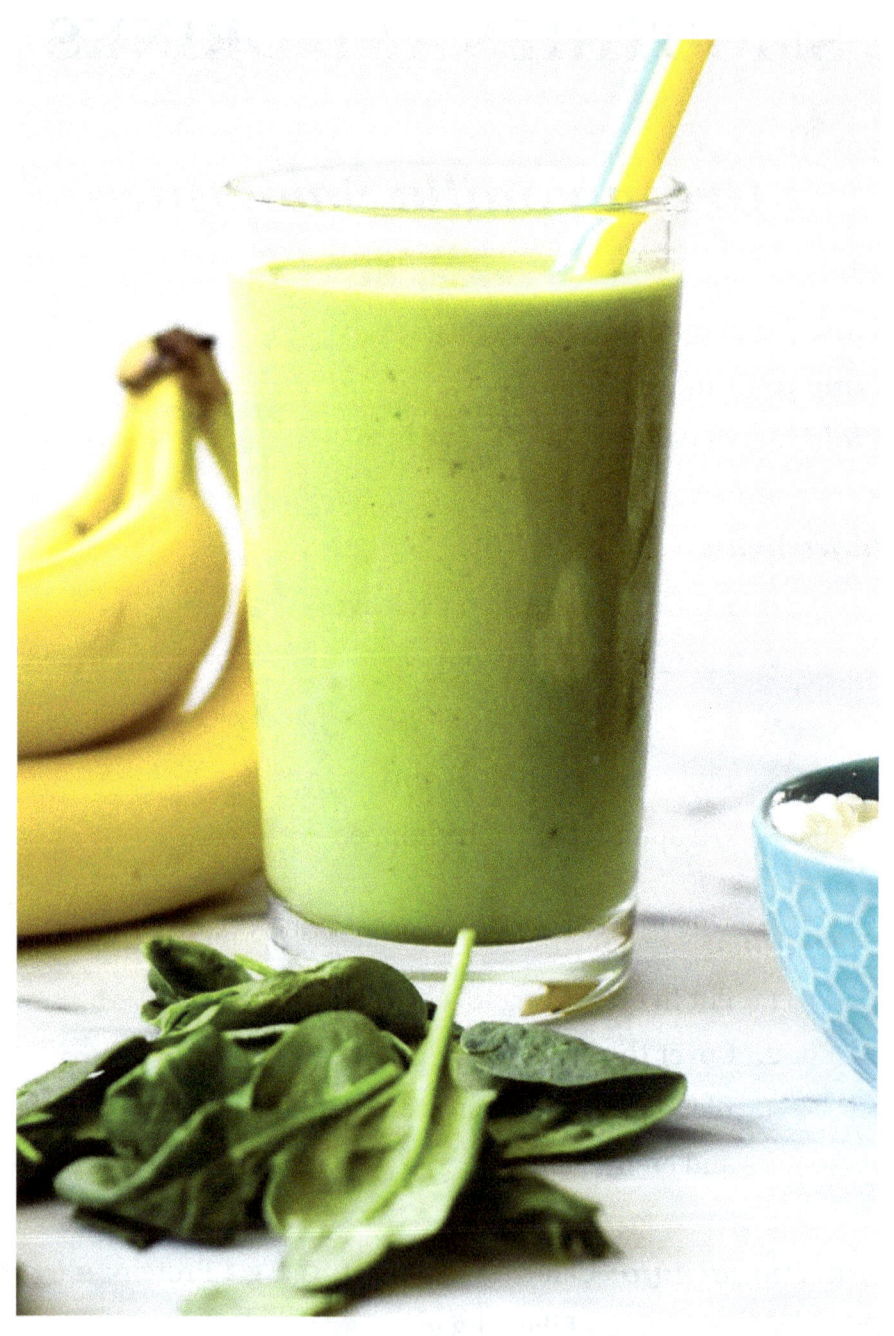

Hibiscus Tea

Time To Prepare: five minutes
Time to Cook: ten minutes
Yield: Servings 4

Ingredients:

- 1 tbsp. honey
- 1 tsp fresh ginger, grated
- 10 cups water
- 2 cup dried hibiscus petals
- Rind from 1 pineapple

Directions:

1. Wash hibiscus leaves meticulously with cold water.
2. Take away the dust.
3. Put in water, honey, and ginger to the instant pot. Stir.
4. Mix in hibiscus petals and pineapple rind.
5. Secure the lid. Cook on HIGH pressure ten minutes.
6. When done, depressurize naturally.
7. Remove pineapple rind. Pass liquid through a fine-mesh strainer.
8. Cool thoroughly. Chill before you serve.

Nutritional Info: Calories: 114 ‖ Fat: 0g ‖ Carbohydrates: 28g ‖ Protein: 0g

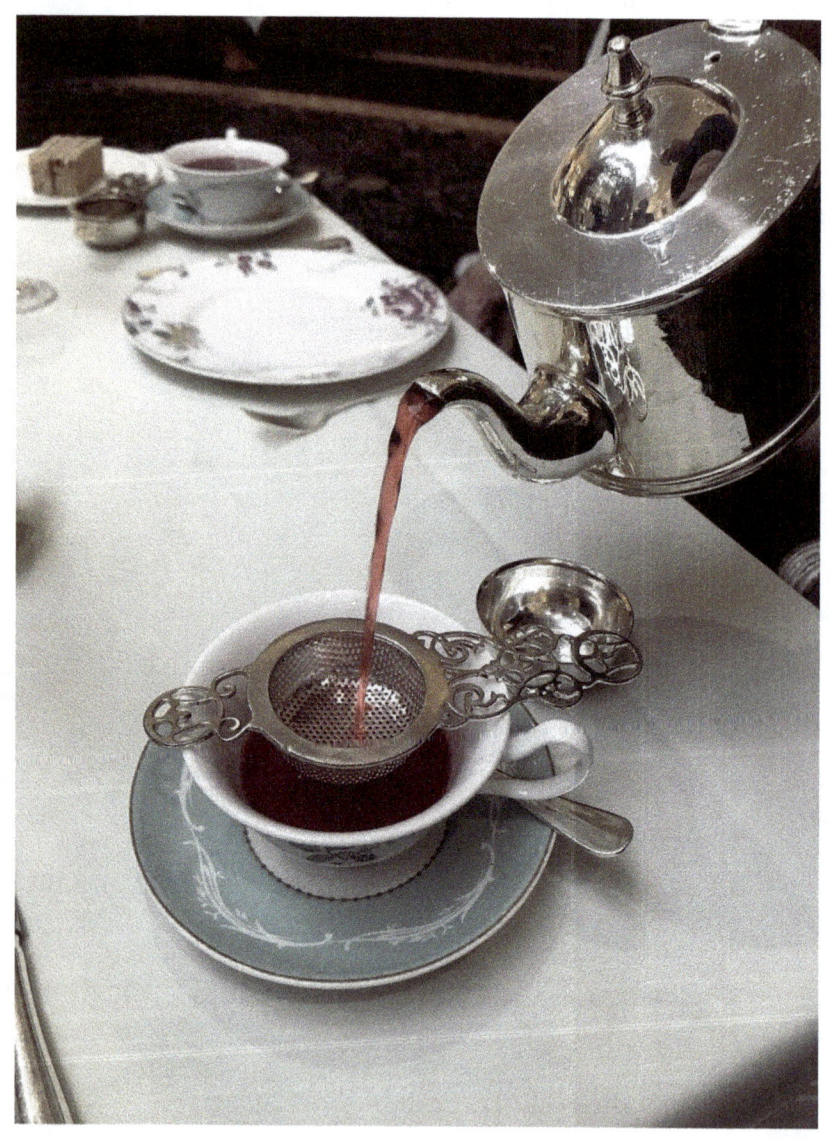

Hot Apple Cider

Time To Prepare: five minutes
Time to Cook: fifteen minutes
Yield: Servings 4

Ingredients:

- ½ cup fresh cranberries
- ½ cup honey
- ½ star of anise
- ½ tsp whole cloves
- 1 lemon, peeled, cut into segments
- 1 orange, peeled, cut into segments
- 2 cinnamon sticks
- 7 medium apples, cored, quarter
- Water to cover ingredients

Directions:

1. Put in apples, lemon, orange, and cranberries to the instant pot.
2. Put in cinnamon stick, star anise, and cloves.
3. Pour in water to immerse ingredients.
4. Secure the lid. Cook on HIGH pressure fifteen minutes.

5. Depressurize naturally.
6. Mash fruit using a masher to release juices.
7. Strain the liquid. Chill completely before you serve.

Nutritional Info: Calories: 153 ‖ Fat: 9g ‖ Carbohydrates: 14g ‖ Protein: 4g

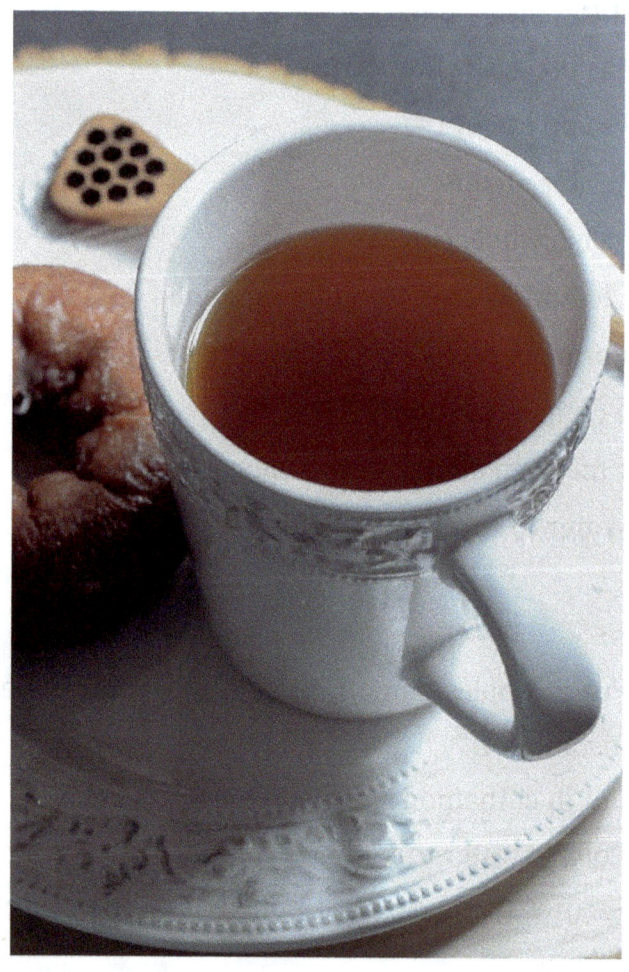

Hot Peppermint Vanilla Latte

Time To Prepare: five minutes
Time to Cook: five minutes
Yield: Servings 4

Ingredients:
- ¼ cup honey
- 1 tsp vanilla
- 2 cups coffee
- 23 drops peppermint oil
- 4 cups almond milk

Directions:
1. Put in listed ingredients to the instant pot.
2. Secure the lid. Cook on HIGH pressure five minutes.
3. When done, depressurize naturally.
4. Serve warm.

Nutritional Info: Calories: 279 ‖ Fat: 3g ‖ Carbohydrates: 61g ‖ Protein: 3g

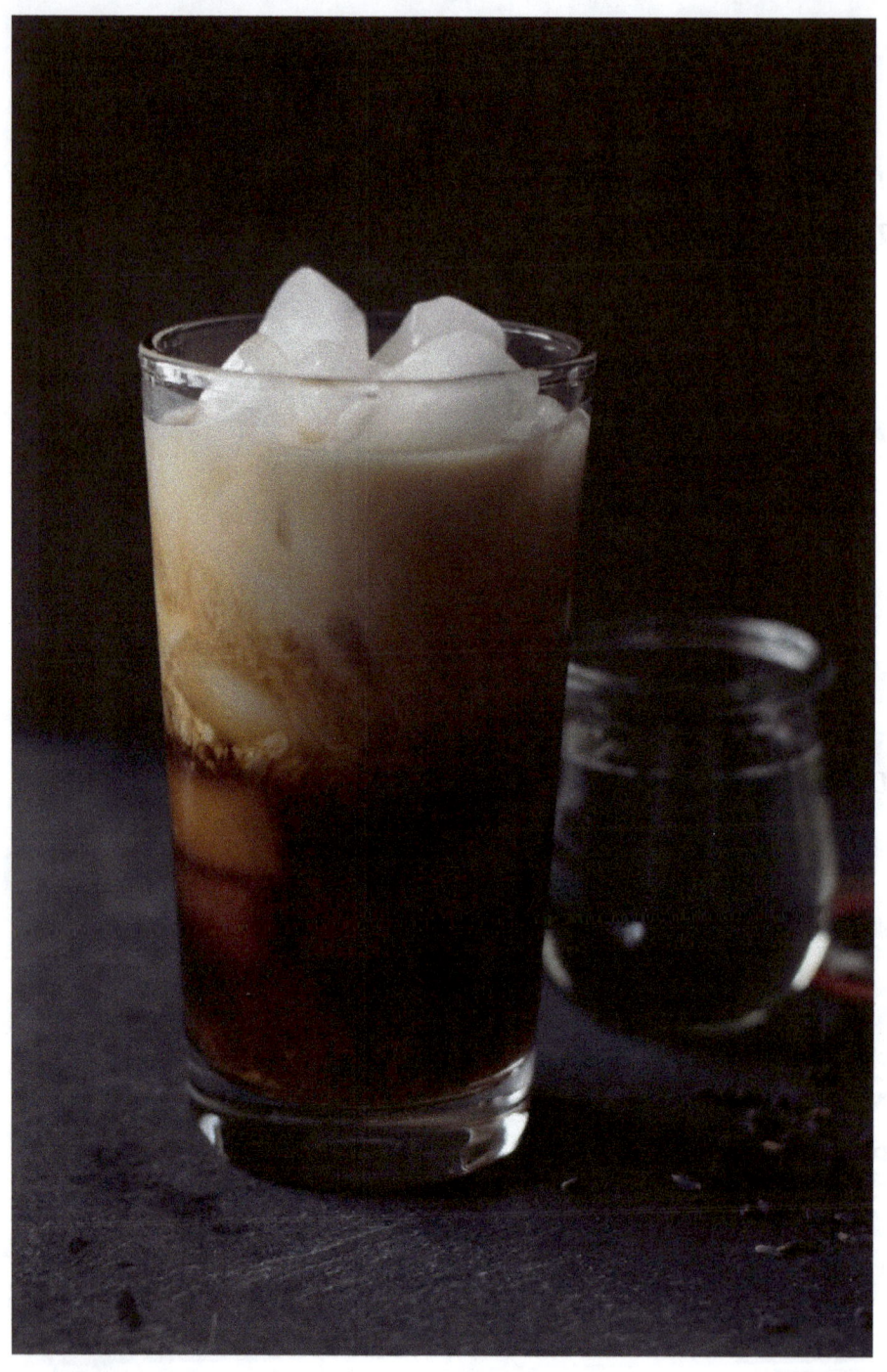

Instant Horchata

Time To Prepare: five minutes
Time to Cook: five minutes
Yield: Servings 4

Ingredients:

- 1 cinnamon stick, broken into little chunks
- 32 ounces rice milk
- 6 tbsp. honey

Directions:

1. Put in listed ingredients to the instant pot.
2. Secure the lid. Cook on HIGH pressure five minutes.
3. When done, depressurize naturally over ten minutes.
4. Cool thoroughly. Chill before you serve.

Nutritional Info: Calories: 226 ‖ Fat: 1g ‖ Carbohydrates: 53g ‖ Protein: 2g

Jamaican Hibiscus Tea

Time To Prepare: five minutes
Time to Cook: five minutes
Yield: Servings 4

Ingredients:

- ½ tsp ginger, minced
- 1 cup dried hibiscus flowers
- 1 tbsp. honey
- 8 cups water
- Ice as required
- Juice of 1 lime

Directions:

1. Put in hibiscus flowers, water, honey, and ginger to the instant pot.
2. Secure the lid. Cook on HIGH pressure five minutes.
3. When done, depressurize naturally.
4. Cool thoroughly. Move to glass decanter. Mix in lime Juice. Pour over ice.

Nutritional Info: Calories: 197 ‖ Fat: 0g ‖ Carbohydrates: 18g ‖ Protein: 0g

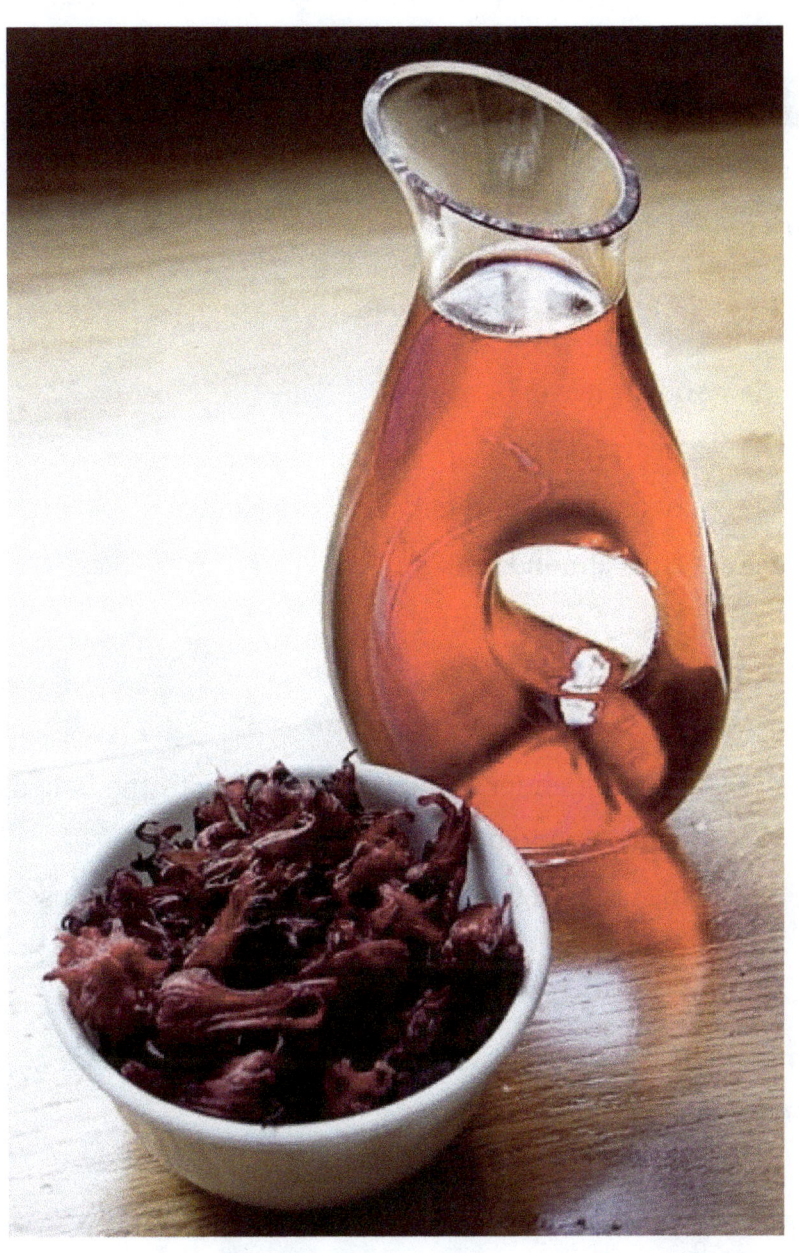

Kale Smoothie

Time To Prepare: ten minutes
Time to Cook: 0 minutes
Yield: Servings 2

Ingredients:

- 10 kale leaves
- 2 pears, chopped
- 5 bananas, peeled and slice into chunks
- 5 cups almond milk
- 5 tbsp. almond butter

Directions:

1. In your blender, combine the kale with the bananas, pears, almond butter, and almond milk.
2. Pulse thoroughly, split into glasses, before you serve. Enjoy!

Nutritional Info: Calories: 267 ‖ Fat: 11 g ‖ Protein: 7 g ‖ Carbohydrates: fifteen g ‖ Fiber: 7 g

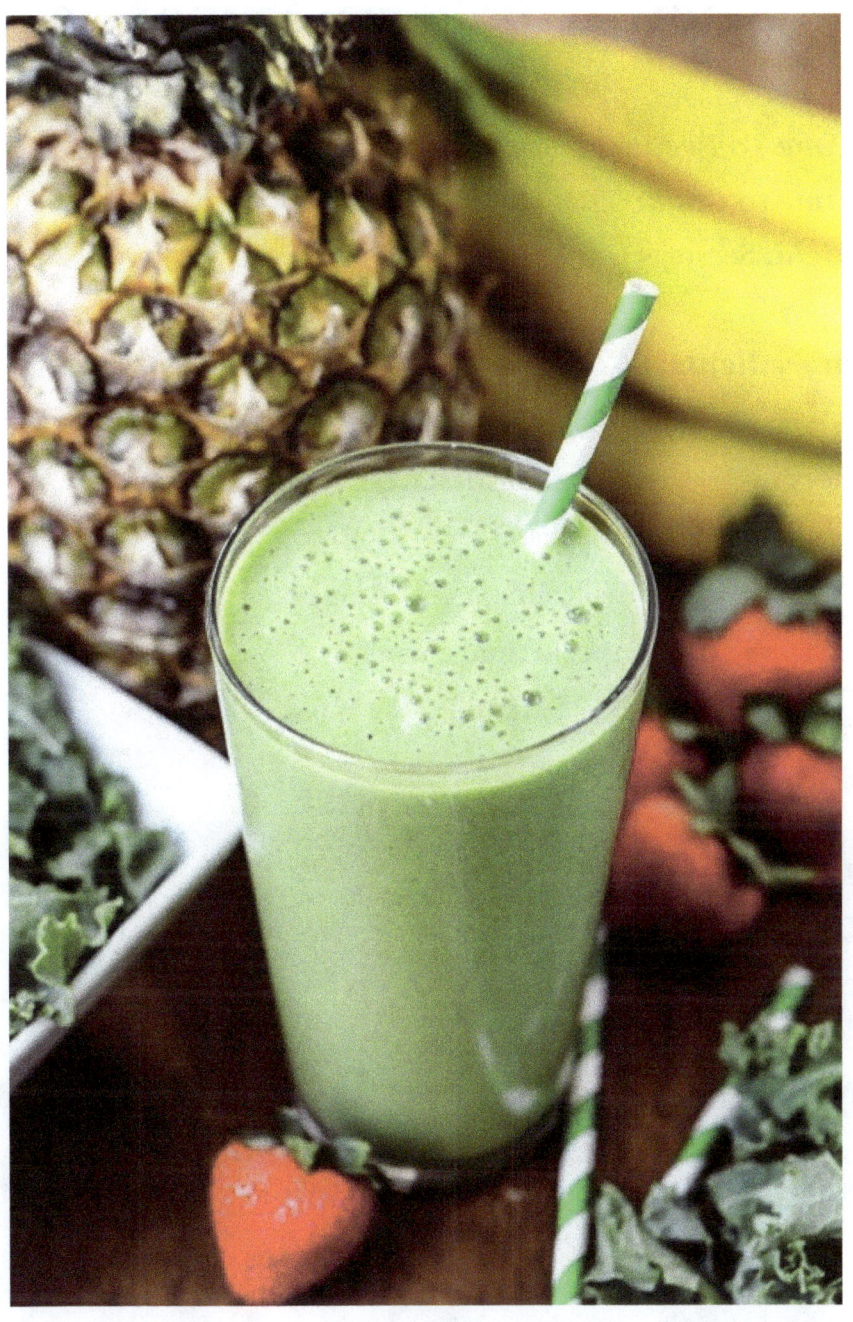

Kiwi Strawberry Smoothie

Time To Prepare: ten minutes
Time to Cook: 0 minutes
Yield: Servings 1

Ingredients:

- ¼ cup Chia seed powder
- ½ cup Strawberries, fresh or frozen, chopped
- 1 Banana, diced
- 1 cup Milk, almond or coconut
- 1 Kiwi, peeled and chopped
- 1 tsp. Basil, ground
- 1 tsp. Turmeric, ground

Directions:

Drink instantly after all the ingredients have been thoroughly combined.

Nutritional Info: Calories 250 ‖ 9.9 grams sugar ‖ 1 gram fat ‖ 34 grams carbs ‖ 4.3 grams fiber ‖

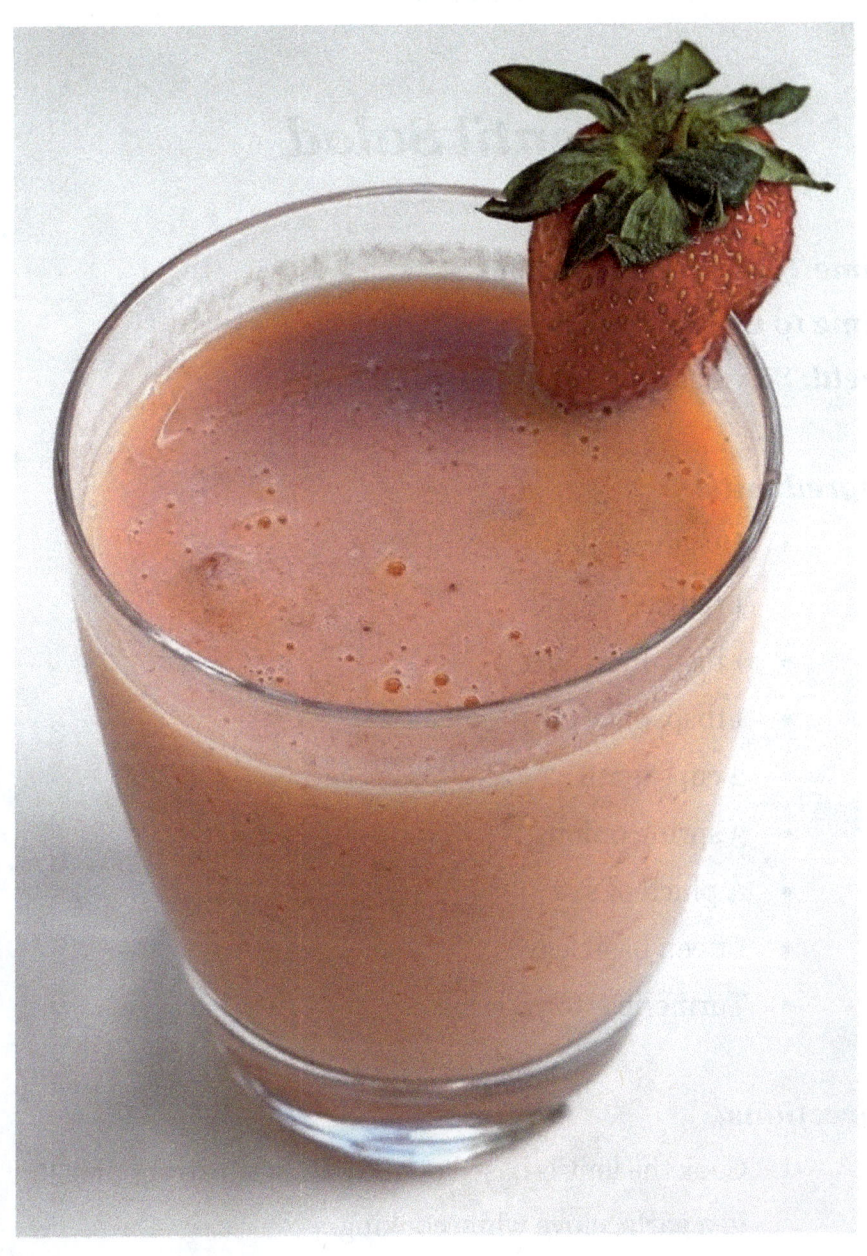

SIDES

Lentil Salad

Time To Prepare: ten minutes
Time to Cook: 0 minutes
Yield: Servings 2

Ingredients:

- ½ cup parsley
- 1 red bell pepper
- 1 tbsp. lime juice
- 1 tbsp. olive oil
- 2 cups lentil
- 3 spring onions
- A pinch of salt
- fifteen basil leaves
- Turmeric – to your taste

Directions:

1. Cook the lentils based on the package instructions. Put in a garlic clove while cooking.
2. When cooled, remove the garlic clove and put the lentils into a big container.

3. Chop all the vegetables then put in them to the lentils.
4. Put in lime juice, a small amount of salt, and olive oil.
5. Mix thoroughly.

Nutritional Info: ‖ Calories: 207 kcal ‖ Protein: 11.53 g ‖ Fat: 10.49 g ‖ Carbohydrates: 22.37 g

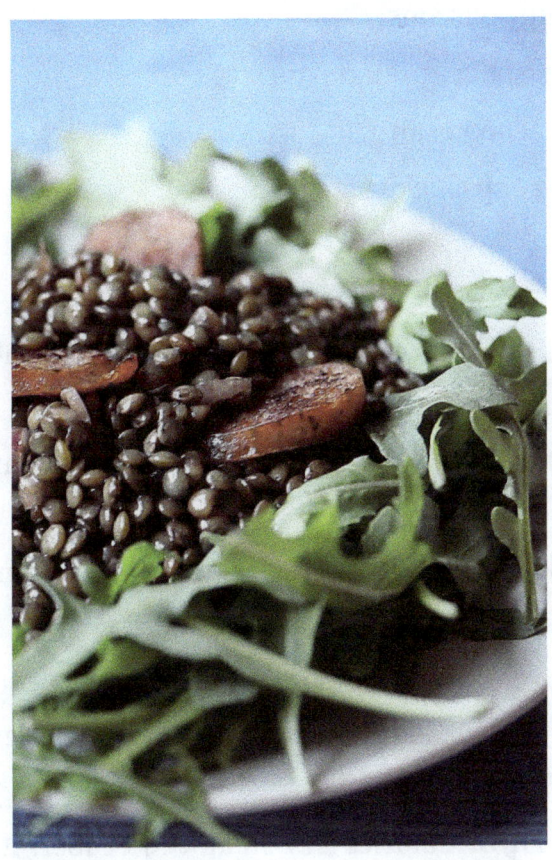

Mascarpone Couscous

Time To Prepare: fifteen minutes
Time to Cook: 7.5 hours
Yield: Servings 4

Ingredients:

- ½ cup mascarpone
- 1 cup couscous
- 1 teaspoon ground paprika
- 1 teaspoon salt
- 3 ½ cup chicken stock

Directions:

1. Put chicken stock and mascarpone in the pan and bring the liquid to boil.
2. Put in salt and ground paprika. Stir gently and simmer for a minute.
3. Take off the liquid from the heat and put in couscous. Stir thoroughly and close the lid.
4. Leave couscous for about ten minutes.
5. Mix the cooked side dish well before you serve.

Nutritional Info: Calories 227 ‖ Fat: 4.9 ‖ Fiber: 2.4 ‖ Carbs: 35.4 ‖ Protein: 9.

Moroccan Style Couscous

Time To Prepare: ten minutes
Time to Cook: ten minutes
Yield: Servings 4

Ingredients:

- ½ teaspoon ground cardamom
- ½ teaspoon red pepper
- 1 cup chicken stock
- 1 cup yellow couscous
- 1 tablespoon butter
- 1 teaspoon salt

Directions:

1. Toss butter in the pan and melt it.
2. Put in couscous and roast it for a minute over the high heat.
3. Then put in ground cardamom, salt, and red pepper. Stir it well.
4. Pour the chicken stock and bring the mixture to boil.
5. Simmer couscous for five minutes with the closed lid.

Nutritional Info: Calories 196 ‖ Fat: 3.4 ‖ Fiber: 2.4 ‖ Carbs: 35 ‖ Protein: 5.9

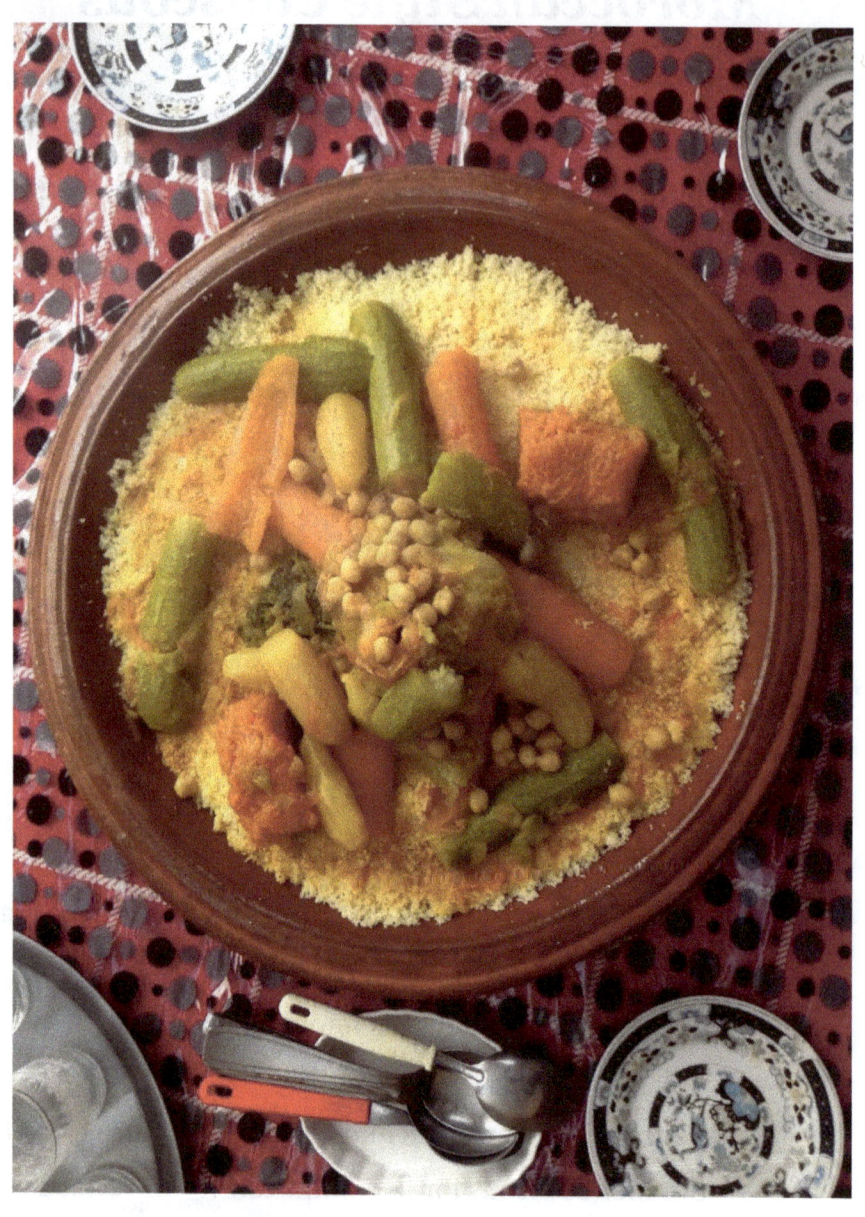

Mushroom Millet

Time To Prepare: ten minutes
Time to Cook: fifteen minutes
Yield: Servings 3
Ingredients:

- ¼ cup mushrooms, cut
- ½ cup millet
- ¾ cup onion, diced
- 1 cup of water
- 1 tablespoon olive oil
- 1 teaspoon butter
- 1 teaspoon salt
- 3 tablespoons milk

Directions:

1. Pour olive oil in the frying pan then put the onion.
2. Put in mushrooms and roast the vegetables for about ten minutes over the moderate heat. Stir them occasionally.
3. In the meantime, pour water in the pan.
4. Put in millet and salt.
5. Cook the millet with the closed lid for fifteen minutes over the moderate heat.

6. Then put in the cooked mushroom mixture in the millet.
7. Put in milk and butter. Mix up the millet well.

Nutritional Info: Calories 198 ‖ Fat: 7.7 ‖ Fiber: 3.5 ‖ Carbs: 27.9 ‖ Protein: 4.7

SAUCES AND DRESSINGS

Cucumber and Dill Sauce

Time To Prepare: ten minutes
Time to Cook: 0 minutes
Yield: Servings 2-4

Ingredients:

- ¼ cup of lemon juice
- 1 cucumber, peeled and squeezed to remove surplus liquid
- 1 cup of freshly chopped dill
- 1 tsp of sea salt
- 450g of Greek yogurt

Directions:

1. In a moderate-sized container, put together the yogurt, cucumber, and dill then stir until well blended. Put in in the lemon juice and salt to taste.
2. Cover and place in your fridge for approximately 1-2 hours before you serve to keep its freshness. Best serve with Mediterranean food, chips, fish, or even bread.

Nutritional Info: ‖ Calories: 97 kcal ‖ Protein: 13.49 g ‖ Fat: 2.1 g ‖ Carbohydrates: 6.34 g

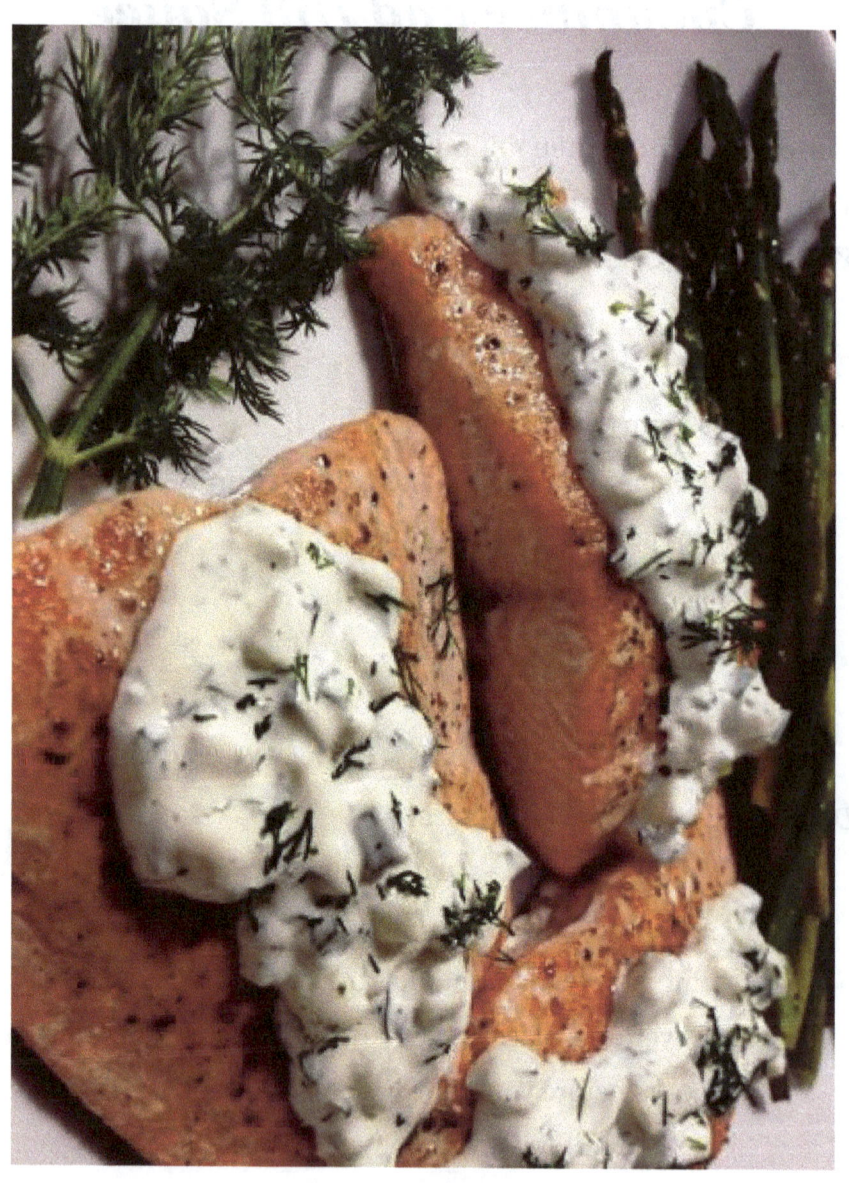

Dairy-Free Creamy Turmeric Dressing

Time To Prepare: ten minutes
Time to Cook: 0 minutes
Yield: Servings 2-4

Ingredients:

- ½ cup of extra-virgin olive oil
- ½ cup of tahini
- 1 tbsp. of turmeric powder
- 2 tbsp. of lemon juice
- 2 tsp of honey
- Some sea salt and pepper

Directions:

1. In a container, whisk all ingredients until well blended.
2. Store in a mason jar and place in your fridge for maximum 5 days.

Nutritional Info: ‖ Calories: 328 kcal ‖ Protein: 7.3 g ‖ Fat: 29.36 g ‖ Carbohydrates: 12.43 g

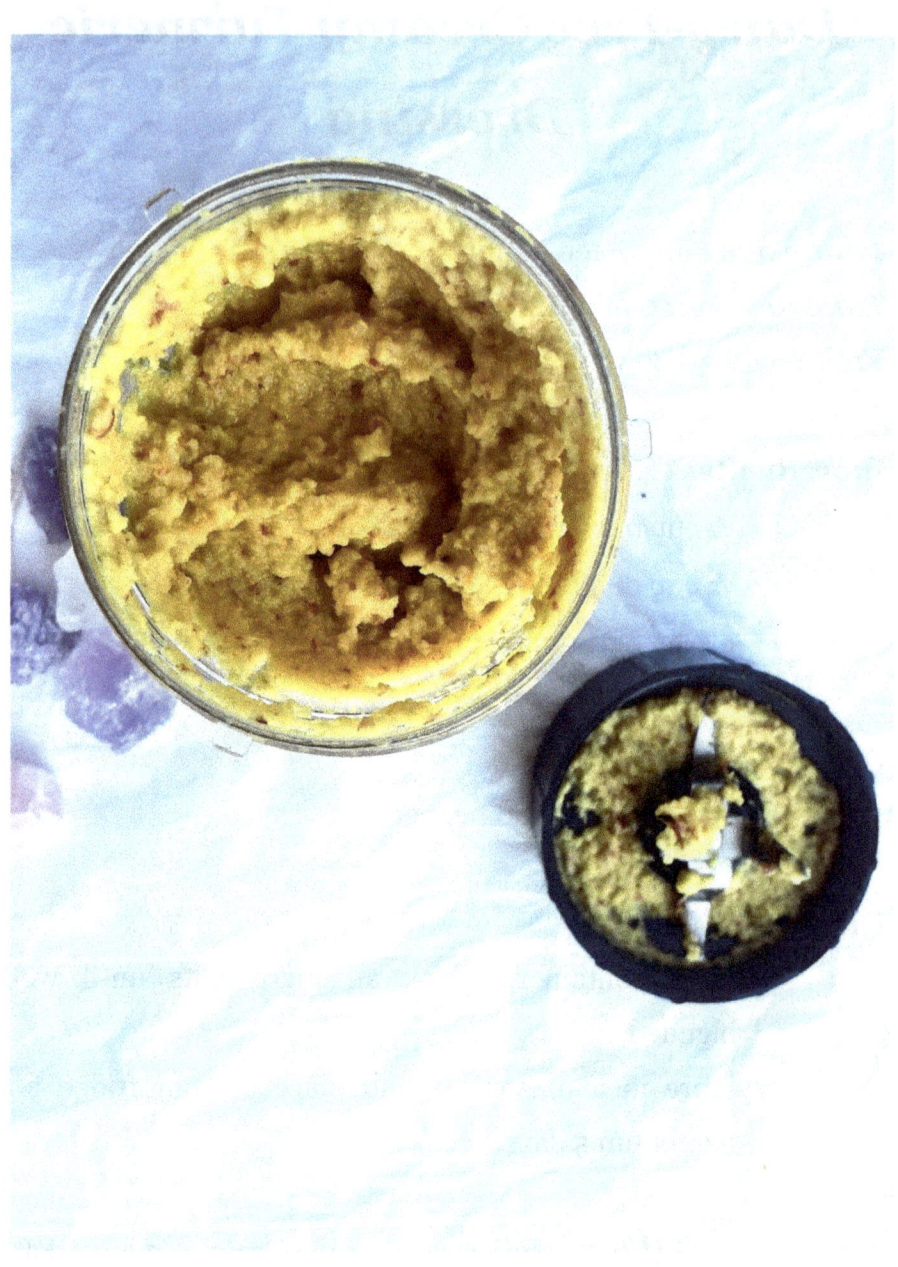

SNACKS

Cottage Cheese with Apple Sauce

Time To Prepare: five minutes
Time to Cook: 0 minutes
Yield: Servings 2

Ingredients:

- ½ teaspoon cinnamon powder
- 5-6 tablespoons cottage cheese
- two to three tablespoons applesauce or more if required

Directions:

1. Split the cottage cheese into 2 bowls.
2. Spread applesauce over the cottage cheese.
3. Drizzle ¼ teaspoon cinnamon powder on each before you serve.

Nutritional Info: ‖ Calories: 79 kcal ‖ Protein: 8.09 g ‖ Fat: 3.45 g ‖ Carbohydrates: 3.92 g

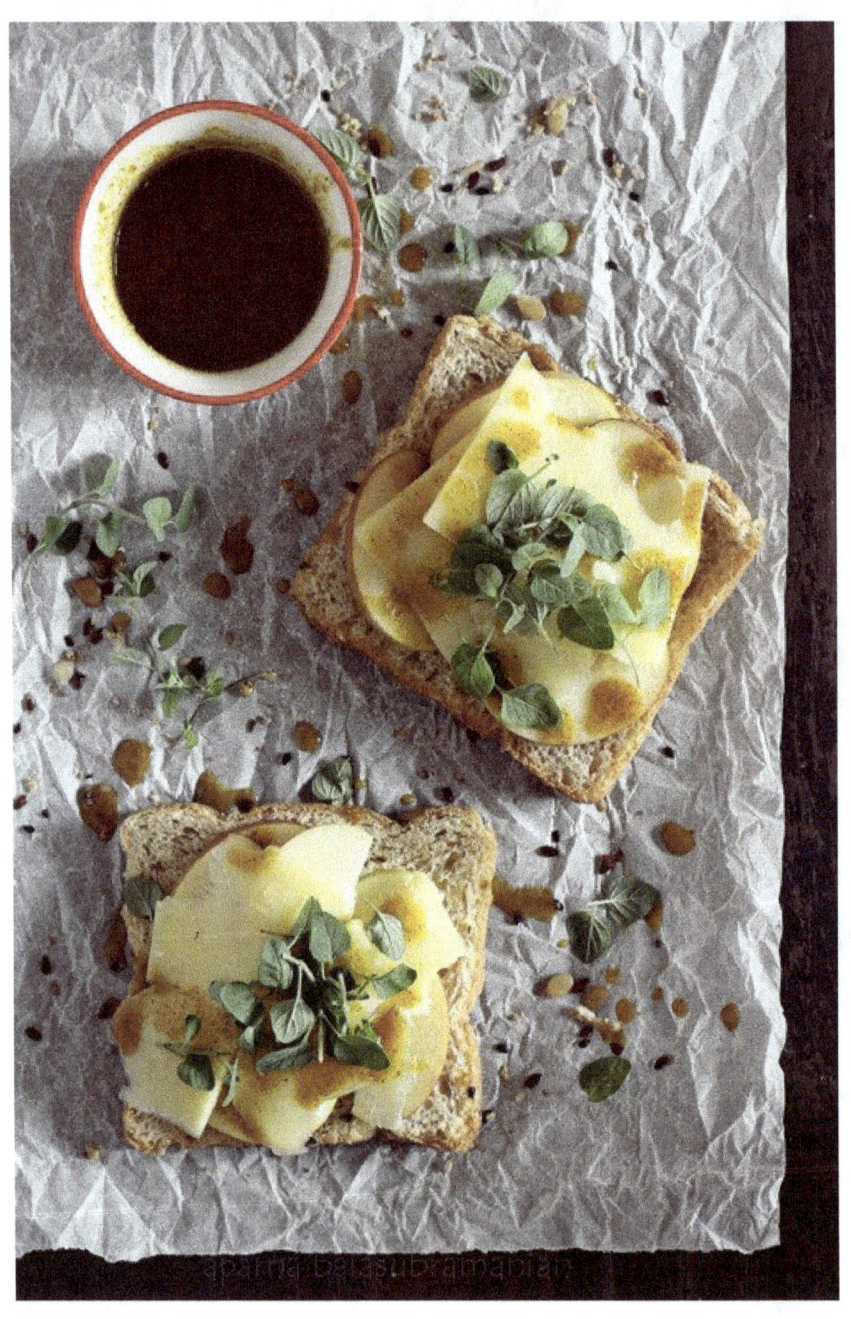

Cucumber Rolls Hors D'oeuvres

Time To Prepare: twenty minutes
Time to Cook: 0 minutes
Yield: Servings 8-10

Ingredients:

- ¼ cup fresh dill, finely chopped
- ½ cup capers
- ½ cup fresh parsley + extra to decorate, finely chopped
- 1 teaspoon Himalayan pink salt
- 2 big organic English cucumbers or 4 normal cucumbers
- 5-6 ripe avocadoes, peeled, pitted, mashed
- For the avocado spread:
- Freshly cracked pepper to taste

Directions:

1. Peel the cucumbers and cut thin slices along the length on a mandolin slicer.
2. Put the cucumber slices on your countertop.
3. To make the avocado spread: Put in all the ingredients of avocado spread into a container and stir until well blended.

4. Spread the avocado mixture uniformly and thinly on the cucumber slices.
5. Begin rolling from one of the shorter ends to the other end and place on a serving platter with its seam side facing down.
6. Repeat the above step with the rest of the cucumber slices.
7. Serve instantly as the cucumbers tend to get soggy after a while.

Nutritional Info: ‖ Calories: 227 kcal ‖ Protein: 3.77 g ‖ Fat: 19.88 g ‖ Carbohydrates: 12.99 g

Cucumber Yogurt

Time To Prepare: five minutes
Time to Cook: 0 minutes
Yield: Servings 1

Ingredients:

- 1 cup cucumbers, skin removed and chopped in chunks
- 1 teaspoon fresh dill, chopped fine
- 1/4 cup fat-free Greek yogurt
- 2 tablespoons chopped cashews
- 2 teaspoons fresh-squeezed lemon juice

Directions:

1. Peel and cut the cucumbers, then put them in a container.
2. Put in the cashews, yogurt, lemon juice, and dill.
3. Mix thoroughly, grab a spoon, and enjoy.

Nutritional Info: ‖ Calories: 300 kcal ‖ Protein: 11.35 g ‖ Fat: 23.55 g ‖ Carbohydrates: 14.13 g

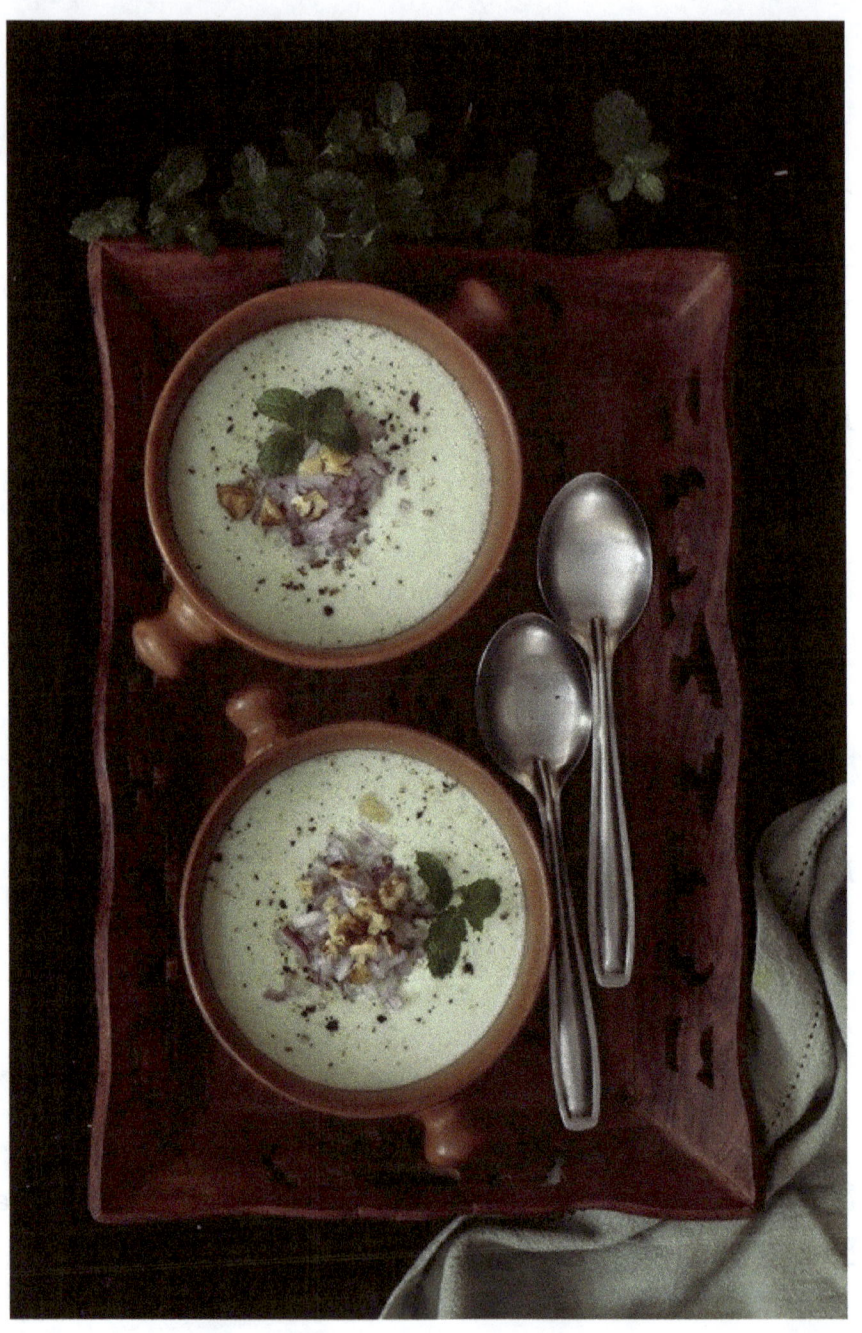

Delectable Cookies

Time To Prepare: twenty minutes
Time to Cook: fifteen-twenty minutes
Yield: Servings 6

Ingredients:

- 1 cup of almonds
- ¼ cup of arrowroot flour
- 1 tbsp. of coconut flour
- 1 tsp. ground turmeric
- Salt, to taste
- Freshly ground black pepper, to taste
- 1 organic egg
- ¼ cup of olive oil
- 3 tbsp. of raw honey
- 1 tsp. of organic vanilla extract
- 1 1/3 cups of almond flour

Directions:

1. Use a food processor to put the almonds and pulse till chopped roughly
2. Move the chopped almonds in a big container.
3. Place the flours and spices and mix thoroughly.

4. In another container, put the rest of the ingredients then beat till well blended.
5. Put the flour mixture into the egg mixture and mix till well blended.
6. Position a plastic wrap over the cutting board.
7. Put the dough over the cutting board.
8. Use your hands to pat into approximately 1-inch thick circle.
9. Gently chop the circle in 6 wedges.
10. Set the scones onto a cookie sheet in a single layer.
11. Bake for approximately fifteen-20 minutes.

Nutritional Info: ‖ Calories: 335 ‖ Fat: 27.7g ‖ Carbohydrates: 17.6g ‖ Protein: 9g ‖ Fiber: 4.8g

Dried Dates & Turmeric Truffles

Time To Prepare: fifteen minutes
Time to Cook: 0 minutes
Yield: Servings 4

Ingredients:

- ¼-tsp black pepper
- ⅓-cup walnuts
- ½-cup rolled oats
- ¾-cup dates, pitted
- 1-Tbsp turmeric powder + more for rolling

Directions:

1. Mix in all the ingredients, excluding the dates in a food processor. Blend until meticulously blended.
2. Put in the dates progressively until forming into the dough.
3. Shape and roll balls from the mixture. Roll each ball with the additional turmeric powder until coating fully.
4. Store the truffles in an airtight jar until ready to serve.

Nutritional Info: ‖ Calories: 95 ‖ Fat: 3.1g ‖ Protein: 4.7g ‖ Sodium: 62mg ‖ Total Carbohydrates: 13.8g ‖ Fiber: 2g ‖ Net Carbohydrates: 11.8g

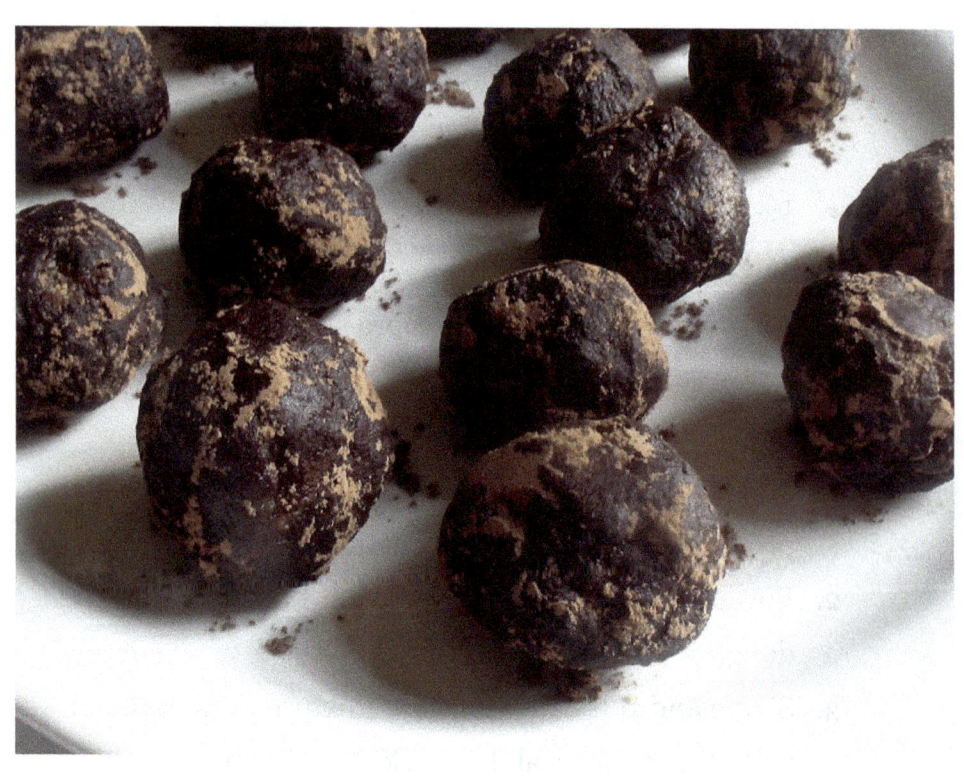

Easy Guacamole

Time To Prepare: ten minutes
Time to Cook: 0 minutes
Yield: Servings 3

Ingredients:
- ½ Teaspoon Sea Salt
- 1 Teaspoon Garlic Powder
- 4 Avocados, Halved & Pitted

Directions:
1. Scoop your avocado flesh out, placing it in a container.
2. Put in in your salt and garlic powder mashing until it's creamy. You can place in your fridge it, and it'll keep for two days.

Nutritional Info: ‖ Calories: 358 ‖ Protein: 7.3 Grams ‖ Fat: 32.2 Grams ‖ Carbohydrates: 13.7 Grams

Easy Peasy Ginger Date

Time To Prepare: twenty minutes
Time to Cook: ten minutes
Yield: Servings 8

Ingredients:

- ¼ cup Almond milk
- ¾ cup Dates
- 1 or 1 ½ cup Almonds or almond flour
- 1 tsp. Ground ginger

Directions:

1. Preheat your oven to 350°F.
2. If you're using fresh almonds, put it through a blender to turn it to almond flour. Blitz for a couple of minutes or so until it looks and feels smooth.
3. Do not blitz for too long, or you might end up making nut butter. Now that you have your almond powder put it in a container and set it aside.
4. Pour the dates and almond milk into your blender and pulse for five minutes. If it doesn't resemble a paste, pulse for another two minutes.
5. Pour in the ground ginger and almond flour. Pulse for three to four minutes to combine.

6. Place the mixture to a baking dish and bake for approximately twenty minutes.
7. Take out of the oven and leave to cool before cutting into bits.
8. Serve or store.

Nutritional Info: ‖ Calories: 55 kcal ‖ Protein: 1.24 g ‖ Fat: 0.99 g ‖ Carbohydrates: 11.24 g

SOUPS AND STEWS

Garlic Mushroom & Beef Soup

Time To Prepare: ten minutes
Time to Cook: forty minutes
Yield: Servings 6

Ingredients:

- ½ cup heavy cream
- ½ cup whipped cream cheese
- 1 pound beef chuck, cubed
- 1 tablespoon coconut oil, for cooking
- 1 yellow onion, chopped
- 1½ cups cremini mushrooms
- 2 cloves garlic, chopped
- 6 cups beef broth
- Salt & pepper, to taste

Directions:

1. Put in the coconut oil to a frying pan and brown the beef.

2. Once cooked, put in the beef to the base of a stockpot with all of the ingredients minus the heavy cream. Mix thoroughly.
3. Heat to a simmer and whisk again until the cream cheese is mixed uniformly into the soup.
4. Cook for half an hour
5. Warm the heavy cream, and then put in to the soup.

Nutritional Info: Calories: 315‖ Carbohydrates: 5g‖ Fiber: 1gNet ‖ Carbohydrates: 4g‖ Fat: 19g‖ Protein: 30g

Garlicky Chicken Soup

Time To Prepare: ten minutes
Time to Cook: fifteen minutes
Yield: Servings 6

Ingredients:

- ¼ teaspoon black pepper
- ½ cup whipped cream cheese
- 1 tablespoon butter for cooking
- 1 teaspoon salt
- 1 teaspoon thyme
- 2 boneless, skinless chicken breasts
- 3 cloves garlic, chopped
- 4 cups chicken broth

Directions:

1. Preheat a stockpot on moderate heat with the butter.
2. Put in the chicken and brown until completely thoroughly cooked. Turn off the heat.
3. Shred the chicken and put in it back to the stockpot together with the rest of the ingredients minus the cream cheese.
4. Heat to a simmer.

5. Put in in the cream cheese and whisk until there are no more clumps.
6. Simmer for about ten minutes before you serve.

Nutritional Info: Calories: 128 ‖ Carbohydrates: 2g ‖ Fiber: 0g Net ‖ Carbohydrates: 2g ‖ Fat: 6g ‖ Protein: 16g

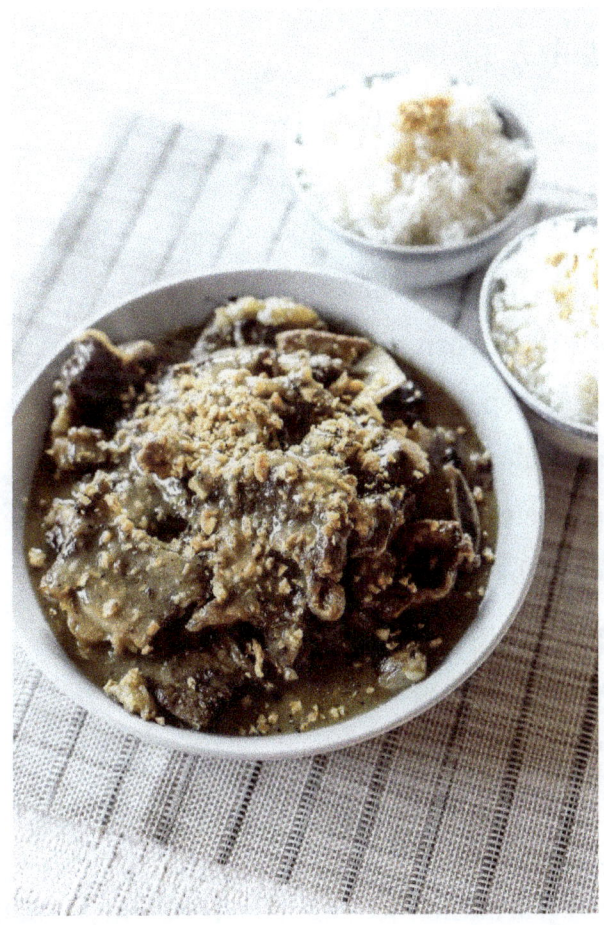

Golden Chickpea And Vegetable Soup

Time To Prepare: fifteen minutes
Time to Cook: twenty minutes
Yield: Servings 6

Ingredients:

- 1 ½ cup Diced celery
- 1 ½ cup Sliced leeks
- 1 cup cooked chickpeas
- 1 cup diced carrots
- 1 cup Torn curly kale leaves
- 1 tbsp. Grated ginger
- 2 cloves minced garlic
- 2 cups Cauliflower florets
- 2 tbsp. Curry powder
- 2 tbsp. Minced organic parsley
- 2 tsp. Coconut oil
- 4 cups Bone broth

Directions:

1. Warm the coconut oil in a pot and put in the garlic and ginger. Sauté for one minute before you put in the

turmeric and curry powder and sautéing for one more minute.
2. Throw in celery, leeks, carrots, and cauliflower, continuously stirring for approximately one minute.
3. Put in the bone broth and chickpeas. Cover the pot and leave to boil. Reduce the heat and allow it to simmer for minimum fifteen minutes.
4. Turn off heat and put in parsley and kale, leaving the heat to cook the leaves.
5. Drizzle salt and pepper.
6. Serve.

Nutritional Info: Calories: 142 kcal ‖ Protein: 8.64 g ‖ Fat: 4.79 g ‖ Carbohydrates: 17.57 g

Greek Split Pea Soup

Time To Prepare: fifteen minutes
Time to Cook: 2 hours
Yield: Servings 6

Ingredients:

- 1 pinch dried marjoram
- 1 potato (diced)
- 1½ pounds ham bone
- 2 onions (cut)
- 2 quarts cold water
- 2-1/4 cups dried split peas
- 3 carrots, (chopped)
- 3 stalks celery (chopped)
- Ground black pepper
- Salt

Directions:

1. Simmer the peas in a pot for a couple of minutes and then soak for an hour.
2. Put in ham bone, onion, marjoram, and seasoning.
3. Boil for 1½ hours.

4. Remove bone and meat. Put in the meat (diced) to the soup.
5. Put the rest of the vegetables and cook until soft.

Nutritional Info: Calories: 310 kcal ‖ Carbohydrates: 58 g ‖ Fat: 20 g ‖ Protein: 2 g

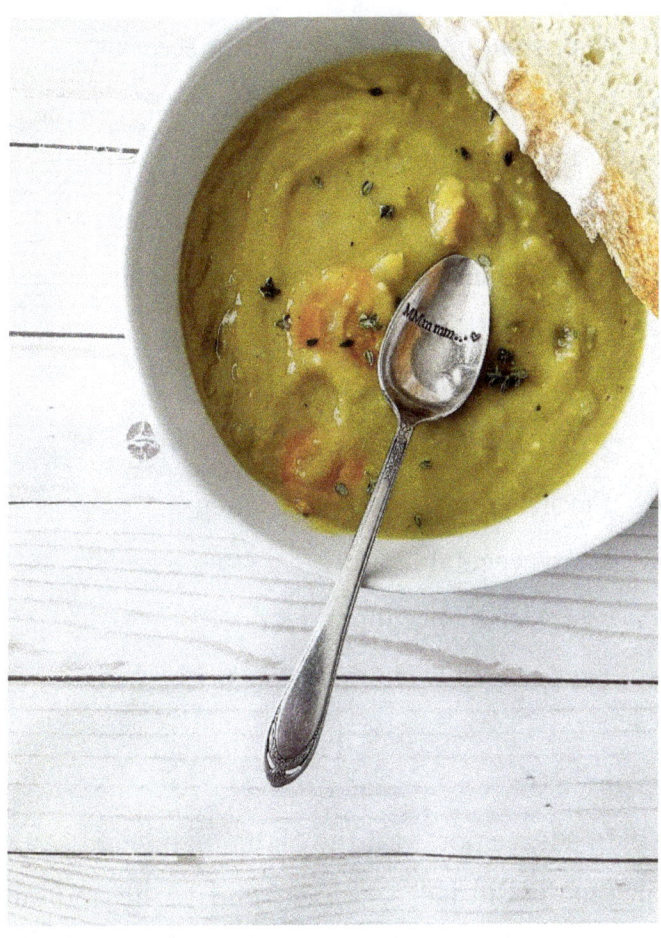

Green Blast Soup

Time To Prepare: ten minutes
Time to Cook: twenty minutes
Yield: Servings 4

Ingredients:

- ¼ cup chopped cashews (not necessary)
- ¼ cup extra-virgin olive oil
- ¼ teaspoon freshly ground black pepper
- 1 bunch Swiss chard, crudely chopped
- 1 fennel bulb, trimmed and thinly cut
- 1 garlic clove, peeled
- 1 teaspoon salt
- 2 leeks, white parts only, thinly cut
- 2 tablespoons apple cider vinegar
- 3 cups vegetable broth
- 4 cups crudely chopped kale
- 4 cups crudely chopped mustard greens

Directions:

1. In a large pot, heat the oil on high heat.
2. Put in the leeks, fennel, and garlic and sauté until tender, for approximately five minutes.

3. Put in the Swiss chard, kale, and mustard greens and sauté until the greens wilt, two to three minutes.
4. Pour the broth then bring to its boiling point.
5. Reduce the heat to a simmer and cook until the vegetables are completely tender and soft about five minutes.
6. Mix in the vinegar, salt, pepper, and cashews (if using).
7. Use an immersion blender to purée the soup in the pot until the desired smoothness is achieved before you serve.

Nutritional Info: Calories: 238 ‖ Total Fat: 14g ‖ Total Carbohydrates: 22g ‖ Sugar: 4g ‖ Fiber: 6g ‖ Protein: 9g ‖ Sodium: 1294mg

Gut-Healing Bone Broth

Time To Prepare: fifteen minutes
Time to Cook: 8 to one day
Yield: Servings 4

Ingredients:

- 1 medium onion, chopped
- 1 tablespoon apple cider vinegar
- 2 bay leaves
- 2 celery stalks, chopped
- 2 pounds beef marrow bones
- 3 medium carrots, chopped
- 4 garlic cloves
- Filtered water, to cover

Directions:

1. In a 6-quart slow cooker, mix the bones, garlic, carrots, celery, onion, bay leaves, and vinegar. Cover with filtered water. Set the cooker on low and simmer for minimum 8 hours and up to one day.
2. Skim off and discard any foam that forms on the surface. Ladle the broth through a fine-mesh sieve or cheesecloth to strain out the solids. Pour into airtight glass containers. The broth can be placed in the fridge

for maximum one week; just boil it again before use. To freeze, let the broth fully cool and then fill jars up to an inch below the top to allow for expansion, and keep for four to 5 months.

Nutritional Info: Calories: 40 ‖ Total Fat: 0g ‖ Saturated Fat: 0g ‖ Cholesterol: 0mg ‖ Carbohydrates: 5g ‖ Fiber: 0g ‖ Protein: 6g

Hamburger & Tomato Soup

Time To Prepare: ten minutes
Time to Cook: 4 hours
Yield: Servings 6
Ingredients:

- ½ cup beef broth
- ½ cup no-sugar added marinara sauce
- ½ cup shredded cheddar cheese
- 1 pound lean ground beef
- 1 yellow onion, chopped
- 2 cloves garlic, chopped
- Salt & pepper, to taste

Directions:

1. Put in all the ingredients to a slow cooker minus the shredded cheese and cook on high for 4 hours.
2. Mix in the cheese before you serve.

Nutritional Info: Calories: 209 ‖ Carbohydrates: 5g ‖ Fiber: 1g Net ‖ Carbohydrates: 4g ‖ Fat: 9g ‖ Protein: 26g

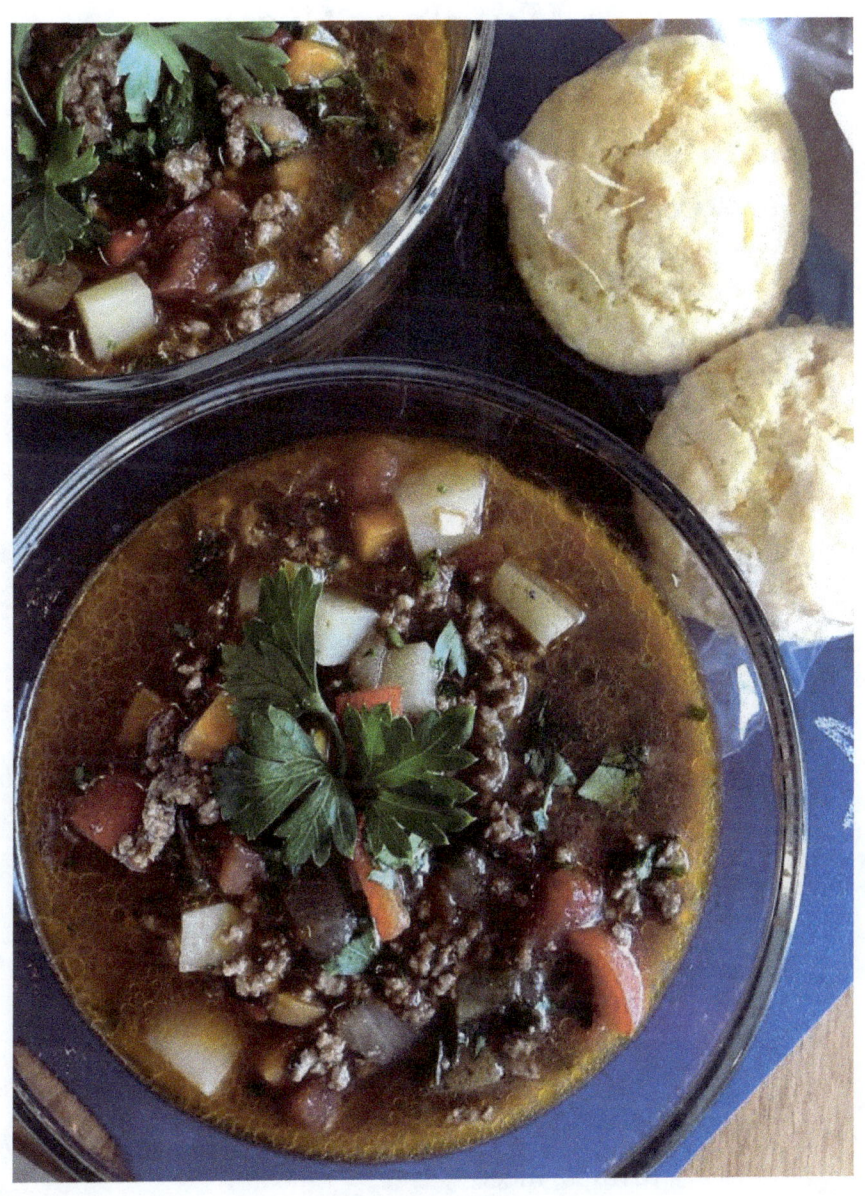

Harvest Stew

Time To Prepare: fifteen minutes
Time to Cook: 60 minutes
Yield: Servings 6

Ingredients:

- ¼ cup flour
- ½ cup cut carrots
- ½ cup diced celery
- ¾ cup diced onions
- 1 bay leaf
- 1 leek, cleaned and diced
- 1 potato, peeled and diced
- 1 pound stewing beef cubes
- 2 cups diced zucchini
- 2 tablespoons olive oil
- 2 tablespoons Worcestershire sauce
- 2 tomatoes, chopped
- 3 sprigs fresh thyme
- 3 turnips, diced
- 4 cups low-sodium beef broth
- 6 garlic cloves, peeled
- Salt and pepper, to taste

Directions:

1. Brown the beef cubes in olive oil. Dust the flour on the meat and stir to coat and spread.
2. Put in the onions, carrots, celery, leek, garlic, zucchini, potato, turnips, tomatoes, bay leaf, thyme sprigs, and beef broth. Put to its boiling point, then reduce the heat and simmer for 60 minutes.
3. Take away the bay leaf and thyme sprigs. Put in the Worcestershire sauce, salt, and pepper. Serve hot.

Nutritional Info: Calories: 254 ‖ Fat: 9.5 g ‖ Protein: 20 g ‖ Sodium: 514 mg ‖ Fiber: 3.5 g ‖ Carbohydrates: 22 g

Hearty Root Vegetable Soup

Time To Prepare: five minutes
Time to Cook: ten minutes
Yield: Servings 4

Ingredients:

- 1 bay leaf
- 1 carrot, cut
- 1 celery, diced
- 1 garlic clove, minced
- 1 parsnip, cut
- 1 tablespoon fresh parsley, roughly chopped
- 1 teaspoon fresh sage
- 2 cups cauliflower, cut into little florets
- 4 cups chicken stock
- 4 tablespoons olive oil
- Kosher salt and freshly ground black pepper, to taste

Directions:

1. Simply drop all of the above ingredients into your Instant Pot.
2. Secure the lid. Choose "Manual" mode and High pressure; cook for about ten minutes. Once cooking is

complete, use a natural pressure release; cautiously remove the lid.
3. Taste, calibrate the seasonings and serve instantly. Enjoy!

Nutritional Info: 190 Calories ‖ 15.6g Fat ‖ 6.1g Total Carbs ‖ 6.7g Protein ‖ 2.6g Sugars

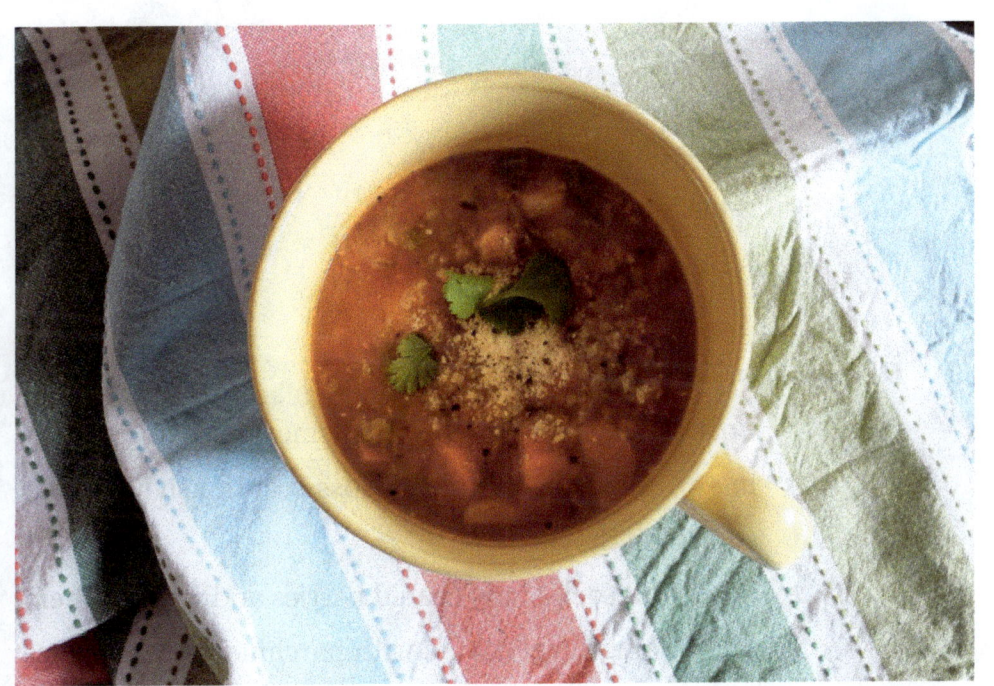

DESSERTS

Creamy & Chilly Blueberry Bites

Time To Prepare: 2 hours and five minutes
Time to Cook: 0 minutes
Yield: Servings 2

Ingredients:

- 1-pint blueberries
- 2-tsp lemon juice
- 8-oz. vanilla yogurt

Directions:

1. Coat the blueberries with the lemon juice and yogurt in a mixing container. Toss cautiously without squishing the berries.
2. Scoop out each of the coated berries and arrange them on a baking sheet coated with parchment paper. Place the sheet in your freezer for a couple of hours before you serve.

Nutritional Info: ‖ Calories: 394 ‖ Fat: 13.1g ‖ Protein: 19.7g ‖ Sodium: 164mg ‖ Total Carbohydrates: 58.9g ‖ Fiber: 9.7g ‖ Net Carbohydrates: 49.2g

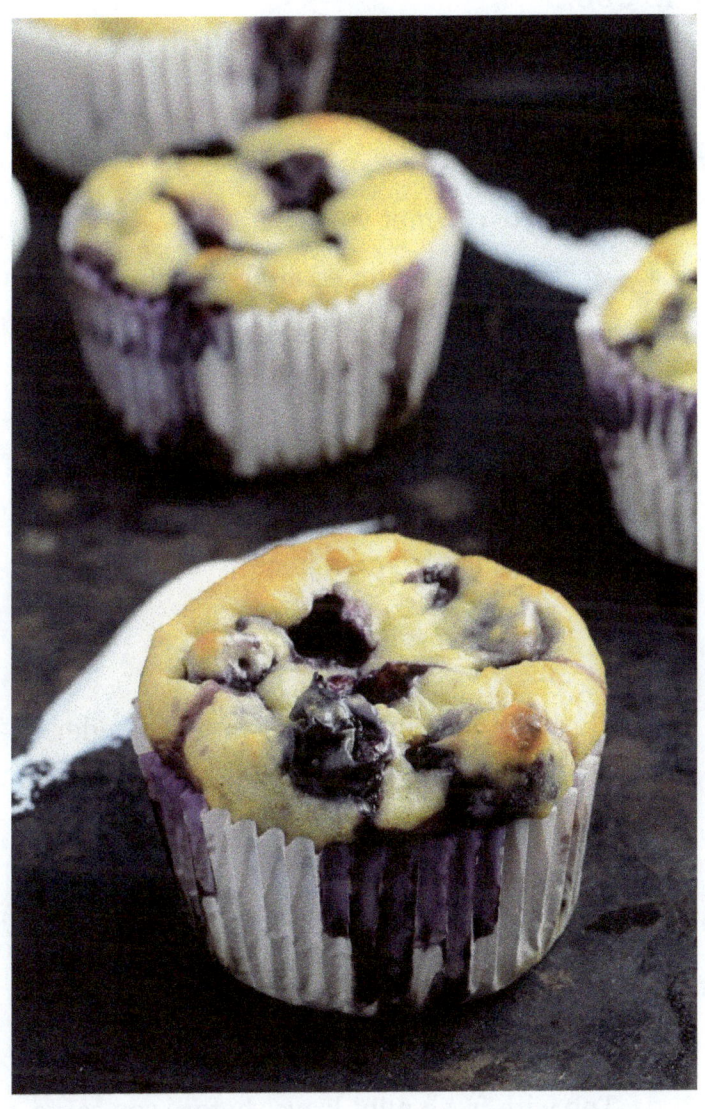

Creamy Frozen Yogurt

Time To Prepare: ten minutes + 2-three hours freezing
Time to Cook:
Yield: Servings 3

Ingredients:

- ½ cup of coconut yogurt
- ½ cup of unsweetened almond milk
- 1 tbsp. of raw honey
- 1 tsp. of fresh mint leaves
- 1 tsp. of organic vanilla extract
- 2 peeled, pitted and chopped medium avocados
- 2 tbsp. of fresh lemon juice

Directions:

1. Throw all the ingredients into a blender apart from mint leaves and pulse till creamy and smooth.
2. Put into an airtight container then freeze for minimum 2-three hours.
3. Take off from the freezer and keep aside for about fifteen minutes.
4. With a spoon stir thoroughly.
5. Top with fresh mint leaves before you serve.

Nutritional Info: ‖ Calories: 105 ‖ Fat: 1.3g ‖ Carbohydrates: 20.3g ‖ Protein: 2.8g ‖ Fiber: 1.4g

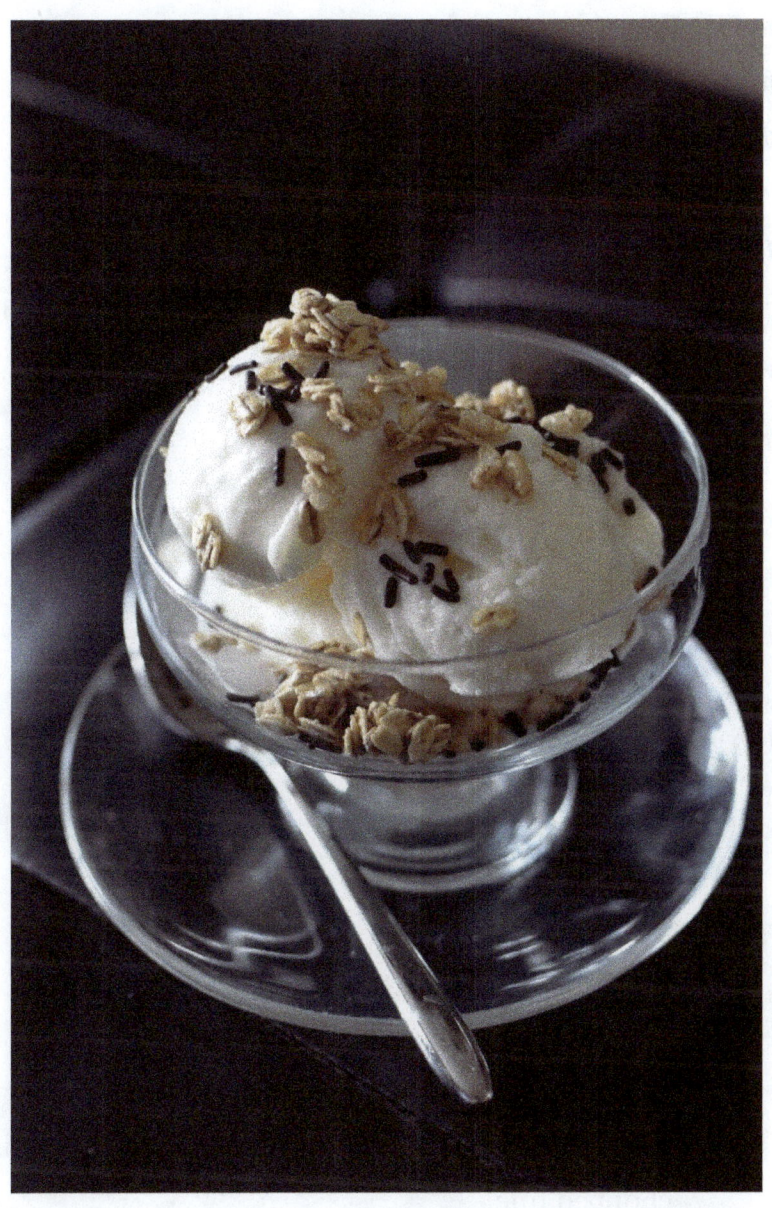

Dark Chocolate Granola Bars

Time To Prepare: ten minutes
Time to Cook: twenty-five minutes
Yield: Servings 12

Ingredients:

- ¼ cup dark cocoa powder
- ¼ cup of flaxseed
- ½ cup dark chocolate chips
- 1 cup of walnuts
- 1 cup tart cherries, dried
- 1 teaspoon of salt
- 1 teaspoon of vanilla
- 2 cups buckwheat
- 2 eggs
- 2/3 cup honey

Directions:

1. Preheat the oven to 350 degrees F.
2. Line with cooking spray your baking pan.
3. Pulse together the walnuts, wheat, tart cherries, salt, and flaxseed in a food processor. Everything must be chopped fine.

4. Mix together the honey, eggs, vanilla, and cocoa powder in a container.
5. Put in the wheat mix to your container. Stir to blend well.
6. Include the chocolate chips. Stir once more.
7. Now pour this mixture into a baking dish.
8. Drizzle some chocolate chips and tart cherries.
9. Bake for about twenty-five minutes. Allow to cool before you serve.

Nutritional Info: Calories 364 ‖ Carbohydrates: 37g ‖ Cholesterol: 60mg ‖ Fat: 20g ‖ Protein: 6g ‖ Sugar: 22g ‖ Fiber: 4g ‖ Sodium: 214mg

Date Dough & Walnut Wafer

Time To Prepare: fifteen minutes
Time to Cook: eighteen minutes
Yield: Servings 8

Ingredients:

- ¼-cup coconut oil
- ¼-tsp sea salt
- ½-cup coconut, unsweetened
- ½-cup walnuts
- ½-tsp baking soda
- ½-tsp sea salt
- 1½-cup oats (divided)
- 18-pcs Medjool dates, pitted
- 1-pc egg
- 1-tsp lemon juice
- 2-Tbsps ground flaxseed
- 6-pcs Medjool dates, pitted and cut into four equivalent portions
- For the Date Layer:

Directions:

1. Preheat the oven to 325°F. Coat a baking pan using parchment paper.

2. Pulse a cup of oats in a food processor until making a flour consistency.
3. Put in in the dates, coconut, baking soda, and sea salt. Pulse again until the dates completely break up.
4. Put in the remaining oats and walnuts, and pulse until the nuts break, but still a bit lumpy. Put in the flaxseed, egg, and oil. Pulse the mixture further until meticulously blended.
5. Set aside ½-cup of the date mixture to use as a topping later. Push down the rest of the mix to a uniform layer in the pan.
6. Wash your food processor, and put in all the date layer ingredients. Pulse the mixture until the dates completely break up and take on a light caramel color.
7. With wet hands, press the mixture down, smoothing it on the date mixture. Crumble and drizzle the reserved date mixture over the top.
8. Place the pan in your oven. Bake for eighteen minutes. Allow the wafer to cool to room temperature before cutting into 16 pieces.

Nutritional Info: ‖ Calories: 203 ‖ Fat: 6.7g ‖ Protein: 10.1g ‖ Sodium: 76mg ‖ Total Carbohydrates: 28.3g ‖ Fiber: 3g ‖ Net Carbohydrates: 25.3g

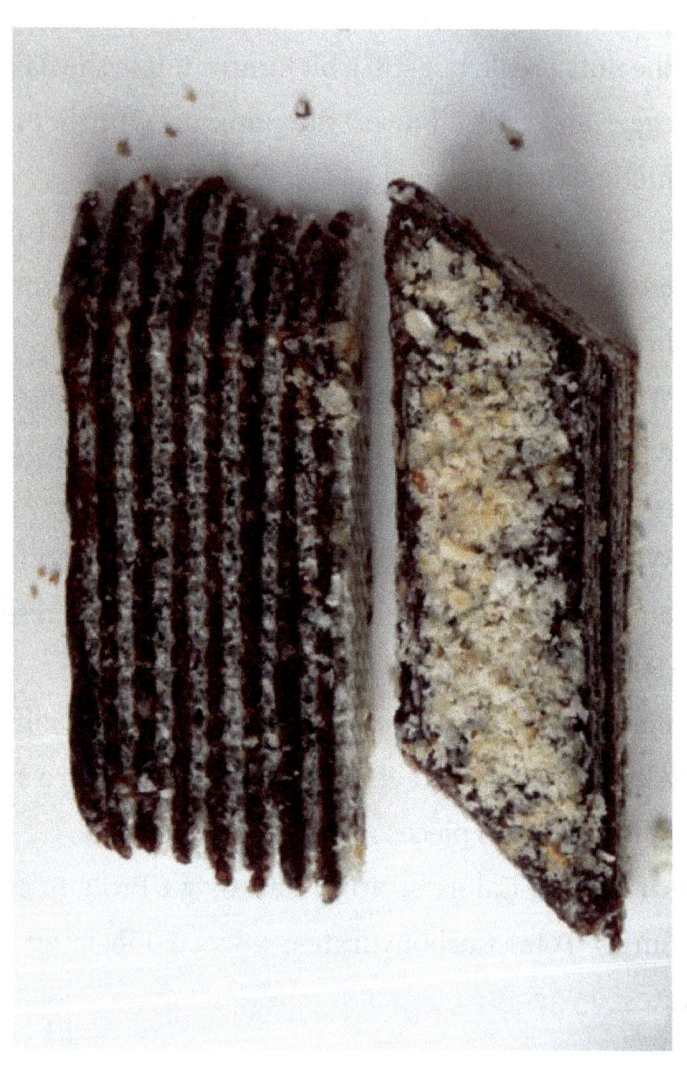

Easy Peach Cobbler

Time To Prepare: five minutes
Time to Cook: twenty minutes
Yield: Servings 6

Ingredients:

- ¼ brown rice flour
- ¼ cup coconut palm sugar, divided
- ¼ cup extra virgin olive oil
- ¼ cup ground flaxseeds
- ½ cup gluten-free oats
- ½ teaspoon cinnamon
- ¾ cup chopped pecans
- 5 organic peaches, pitted and chopped

Directions:

1. Preheat your oven to 350oF.
2. Grease the bottom of 6 ramekins.
3. In a container, combine the peaches, ½ of the coconut sugar, cinnamon, and pecans.
4. Distribute the peach mixture into the ramekins.
5. In the same container, combine the oats, flaxseed, rice flour, and oil. Put in in the rest of the coconut sugar. Mix until a crumbly texture is formed.

6. Top the mixture over the peaches.
7. Put for about twenty minutes.

Nutritional Info: Calories 26 ‖ Fat: 11g ‖ Carbohydrates: 28g ‖ Protein: 10g ‖ Sugar: 12g ‖ Fiber: 6g

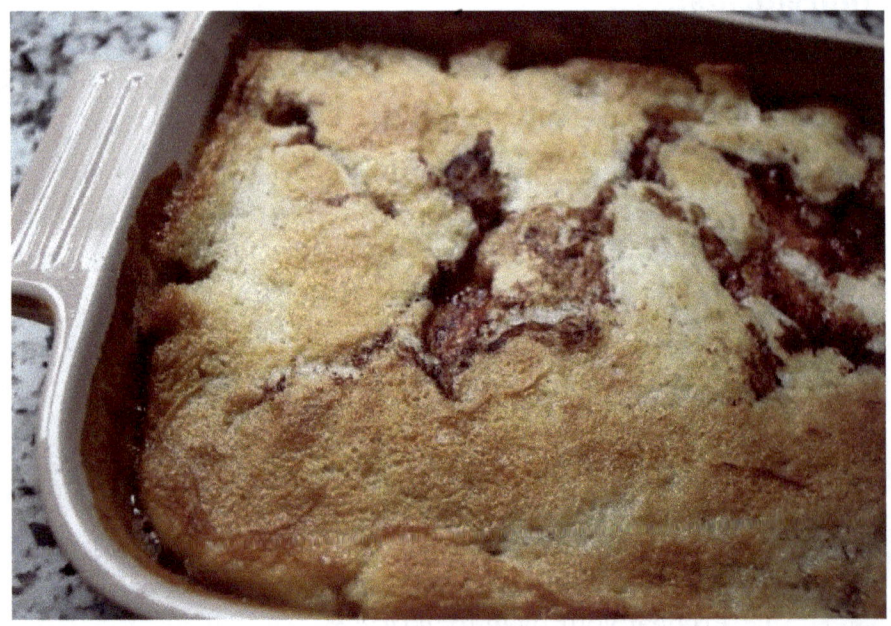

Fall-Time Custard

Time To Prepare: fifteen minutes
Time to Cook: 60 minutes
Yield: Servings 6

Ingredients:

- ¼ tsp. of ground ginger
- 1 cup of canned pumpkin
- 1 cup of coconut milk
- 1 tsp. of ground cinnamon
- 1 tsp. of organic vanilla extract
- 2 organic eggs
- 2 pinches of freshly grated nutmeg
- 8-10 drops of liquid stevia
- Pinch of salt

Directions:

1. Preheat your oven to 350 degrees F.
2. In a big container, put together pumpkin and spices then mix.
3. In another container, put in the eggs and beat thoroughly.

4. Put in the rest of the ingredients then whisk till well blended.
5. Put in egg mixture into pumpkin mixture and mix till well blended.
6. Move the mixture toto 6 ramekins.
7. Position the ramekins in a baking dish,
8. Put in sufficient water in the baking dish about two-inch high around the ramekins.
9. Bake for approximately 1 hour or till a toothpick inserted in the middle comes out clean.

Nutritional Info: ‖ Calories: 131 ‖ Fat: 11.1g ‖ Carbohydrates: 6.1g ‖ Protein: 3.3g ‖ Fiber: 2.3g

Fennel and Almond Bites

Time To Prepare: ten minutes + three hours freezing time
Time to Cook: twenty-five minutes
Yield: Servings 10

Ingredients:

- ¼ cup almond milk
- ¼ cup of cocoa powder
- ½ cup almond oil
- 1 teaspoon fennel seeds
- 1 teaspoon vanilla extract
- A pinch of sunflower seeds

Directions:

1. Take a container and mix the almond oil and almond milk
2. Beat until the desired smoothness is achieved and shiny by using an electric beater

Stir in the remaining ingredients

3. Take a piping bag and pour into a parchment paper-lined baking sheet
4. Freeze for around three hours and stored in your refrigerator

Nutritional Info: ‖ Total Carbohydrates: 1g ‖ Fiber: 1g ‖ Protein: 1g ‖ Fat: 20g

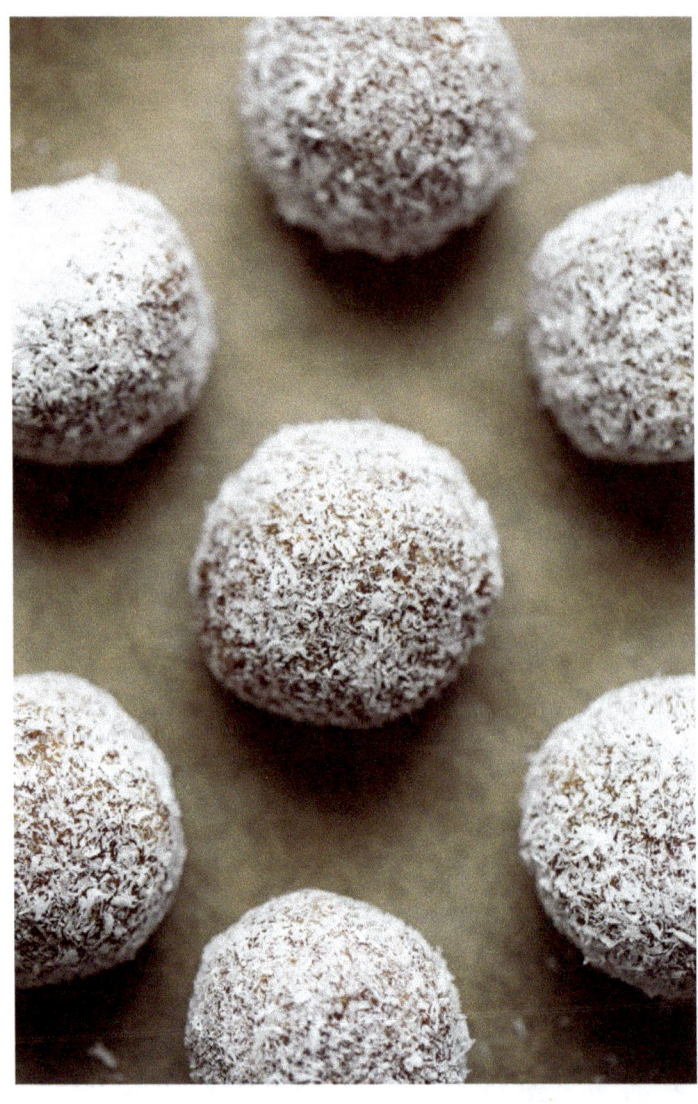

Flourless Sweet Potato Brownies

Time To Prepare: ten minutes
Time to Cook: thirty minutes
Yield: Servings 9

Ingredients:

- ¼ cup Unsweetened Cocoa powder
- ½ cup Almond butter
- ½ cup Cooked sweet potato
- ½ tsp. Baking soda
- 1 big Whole egg
- 2 tsp. Vanilla extract
- 3 tbsp. Dairy-free chocolate chips, optional.
- 6 tbsp. Honey

Directions:

1. Prep the oven by preheating to 350°F.
2. Coat a baking pan using parchment paper leaving a few extra inches on the sides to make it easier to discard or remove
3. Blend all the ingredients, excluding the chocolate chips until you get a super smooth and tender batter.

4. Move the creamy batter to your readied baking pan and use a spatula to spread it around, so it looks almost even.
5. Slide it in your oven, then bake for thirty minutes or until a knife inserted into the pan comes out clean.
6. Remove from the oven and leave to cool in the pan for fifteen minutes before putting it up on a wire rack.
7. If you decide to use the chocolate chip topping, put the chips in a microwave-safe dish and heat until it completely melts. Remove from the microwave and sprinkle over the brownies.
8. Serve or store!

Nutritional Info: ‖ Calories: 171 kcal ‖ Protein: 5.17 g ‖ Fat: 9.28 g ‖ Carbohydrates: 20.01 g

Fried Pineapple Slice

Time To Prepare: ten minutes
Time to Cook: 8 minutes
Yield: Servings 8
Ingredients:

- ¼ cup of coconut oil
- ¼ cup of coconut palm sugar
- ¼ teaspoon of ground cinnamon
- 1 fresh pineapple (peeled and slice into big slices)

Directions:

1. Warm a huge cast-iron frying pan on moderate heat.
2. Put in oil and sugar and cook until the coconut oil has melted while stirring constantly.
3. Put in the pineapple slices into two batches and cook for roughly 1-2 minutes.
4. Flip the medial side and cook for approximately one minute. Carry on cooking for one more minute.
5. Repeat the steps with the rest of the slices.
6. Drizzle with cinnamon before you serve.

Nutritional Info: ‖ Calories: 138 ‖ Fat: 7g ‖ Carbohydrates: 20.9g ‖ Sugar: 15.7g ‖ Protein: 0.6g ‖ Sodium: 15mg

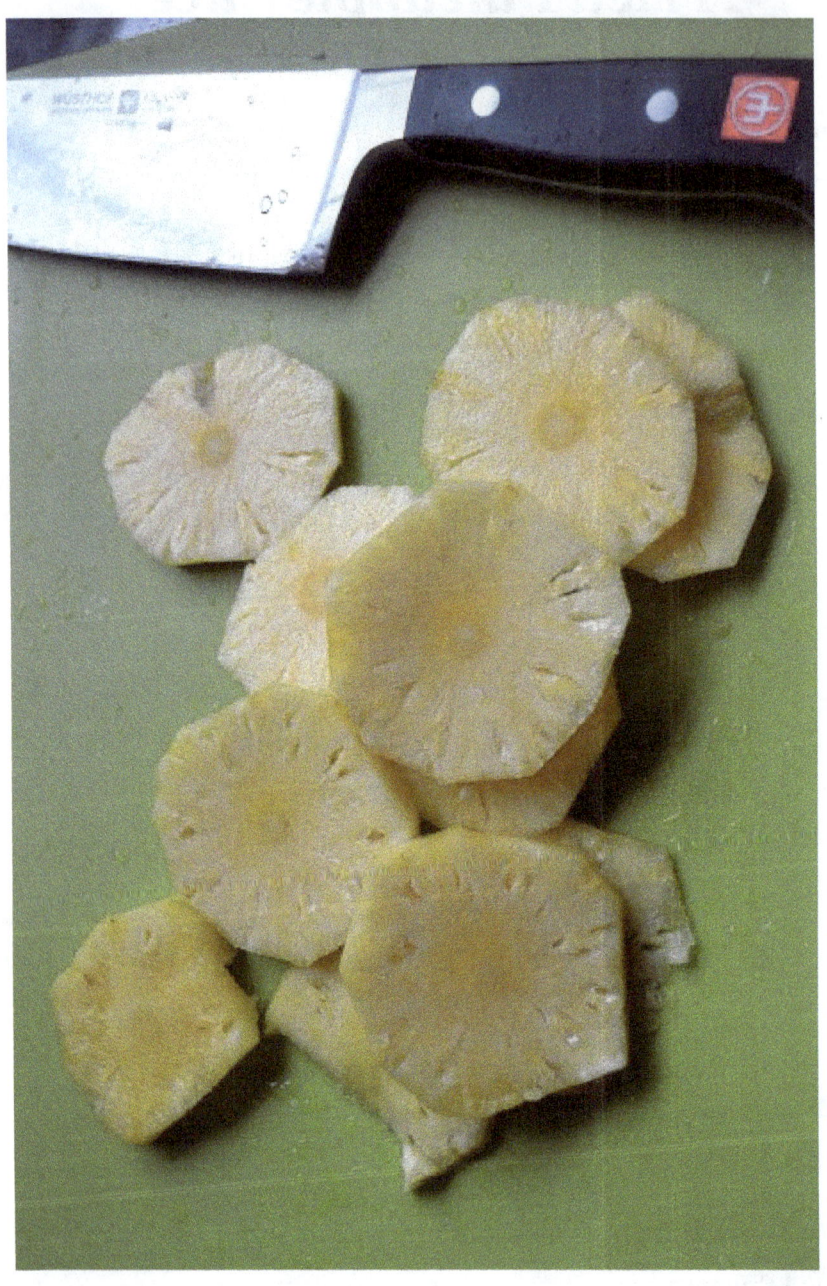

Fruit Cobbler

Time To Prepare: ten minutes
Time to Cook: twenty minutes
Yield: Servings 8

Ingredients:

- ¼ Cup Coconut Oil, Melted
- ¼ Cup Coconut Sugar
- ½ Teaspoon Vanilla Extract, Pure
- ¾ Cup Almond Flour
- ¾ Cup Rolled Oats
- 1 Teaspoon Coconut Oil
- 1 Teaspoon Ground Cinnamon
- 2 Cups Nectarines, Fresh & Sliced
- 2 Cups Peaches, Fresh & Sliced
- 2 Tablespoons Lemon Juice, Fresh
- Dash Salt
- Filter Water for Mixing

Directions:

1. Begin by heating the oven to 425.
2. Get out a cast-iron frying pan, coating it with a teaspoon of coconut oil.

3. Mix your lemon juice, peaches, and nectarines together in the frying pan.
4. Prepare your food processor, mixing your almond flour, oats, coconut sugar, and remaining coconut oil. Put in in your cinnamon, vanilla, and salt, pulsing until the oat mixture looks like a dry dough.
5. If you need more moisture, put in filtered water a tablespoon at a time, and then break the dough into chunks, spreading it across the fruit.
6. Bake for 20 minutes before you serve warm.

Nutritional Info: ‖ Protein: 4 Grams ‖ Fat: 12 Grams ‖ Carbohydrates: fifteen Grams

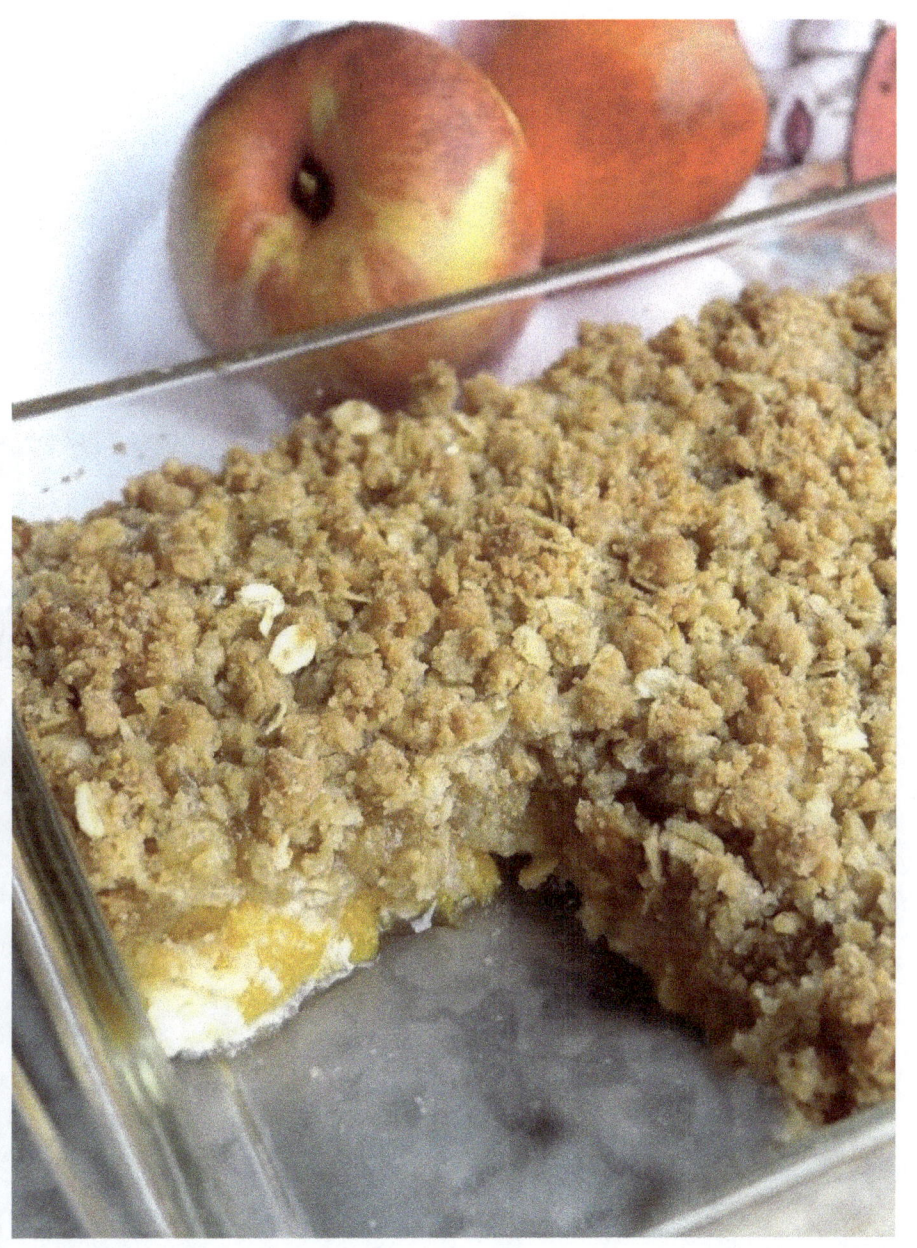

www.ingramcontent.com/pod-product-compliance
Lightning Source LLC
Chambersburg PA
CBHW070734030426
42336CB00013B/1972